Reflexology for Hands and Feet

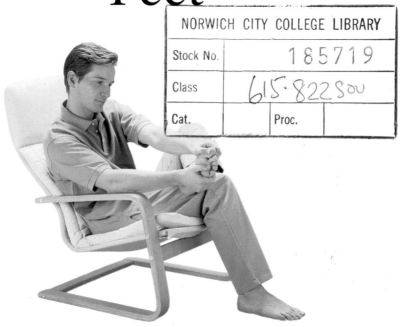

Gillian Soutar

Cert. Ed. MAR MIFA

MARSHALL PUBLISHING • LONDON

A Marshall Edition
Conceived, edited and designed by
Marshall Editions
The Orangery
161 New Bond Street
London W1Y 9PA

First published in the UK in 1999 by
Marshall Publishing Ltd

ISBN: 1-84028-242-8

Originated in Singapore by Chroma Graphics

Printed and bound in Portugal by Printer
Portuguesa.

Project Editor Wendy James

Art Editor Hugh Schermuly

Designer Masumi Higo

Photo stylist Frances de Rees

Managing Editor Anne Yelland

Managing Art Editors Patrick
Carpenter, Helen Spencer

Editorial Director Ellen Dupont

Art Director Dave Goodman

Copy Editor Lindsay McTeague

Editorial Coordinator Becca Clunes

Production Nikki Ingram

Dedication
I dedicate this book to all my family,
especially my husband Dennis and
children Karen and Alastair.

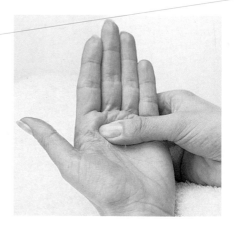

Note
Every effort has been taken to ensure that all
information in this book is correct and
compatible with national standards generally
accepted at the time of publication. This book is
not intended to replace consultation with your
doctor or other healthcare professional. The
author and publisher disclaim any liability, loss,
injury or damage incurred as a consequence,
directly or indirectly, of the use and application
of the contents of this book.

CONTENTS

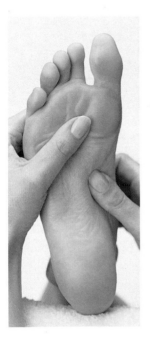

Reproductive system

Cardiovascular system

Lymphatic system

Full foot treatment

Full hand treatment

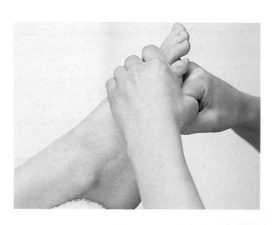

INTRODUCTION

This book is for all who would like to take a natural approach to their health and well being. The practice of reflexology is recognized as a safe and effective way of balancing the body. It helps you relax and encourages the parts of the body to be self healing.

THE HISTORY

Foot and hand reflexology is a form of holistic healing that originated in China 5,000 years ago. It works by stimulating the nerve endings of the feet and hands to bring about a feeling of deep relaxation.

While no written documentation exists to provide a precise history of reflexology, there is a wall painting in an Egyptian tomb at Saqqara which shows four people, two of whom are working on the others' hands and feet. The hieroglyphic inscription on the painting, which has been dated 2330 BC, was translated as "Do not hurt me, I shall act so you praise me".

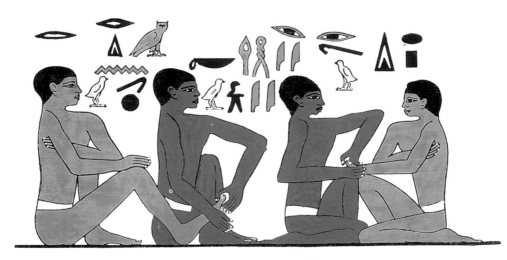

REFLEXOLOGY TODAY

Today's reflexology is attributed to Eunice Ingham, a physiotherapist who had been working with Dr Joe Shelby Riley, a practitioner of zone therapy, a healing system devised in the early years of the 20th century by fellow American William Fitzgerald. In the 1930s she separated the zones from reflexes to show how the feet in particular represented different parts of the body, the right foot representing the right side, the left foot the left side. She then transposed the anatomy of the body to the reflex points of the feet.

Eunice Ingham at first called the therapy compression massage, but eventually changed it to reflexology which, when she took it to the general public, was regarded as witchcraft. She set up a school in the United States to teach others, and now reflexology is practised all over the world. She wrote the first books on the subject. *Stories the Feet Can Tell* and *Stories the Feet Have Told* are about her own experiences and the benefits people gained from her treatments.

THE PHILOSOPHY OF REFLEXOLOGY

Reflexology is the study and practice of working the reflex points of the feet and hands that relate to various parts of the body. It is holistic in approach, taking the whole person, rather than their symptoms or condition, into account. The therapy looks at the person's physical, emotional, mental and environmental factors, working on the principle that the body needs to be balanced on all levels to be fit and healthy. It is a very relaxing form of treatment, encouraging individuals to let go of their negative stresses, to take time for themselves.

Like acupuncture and other eastern therapies, reflexology is based on the theory that good health depends on the on-going flow of energy – "chi" – within the body. This energy needs to flow freely along pathways (meridians or zones) but it can become sluggish through stress, tension, illness and trauma, which in turn can make you feel low and susceptible to illness.

Reflexologists believe that stimulating the main meridians of the feet and hands will unblock the pathways to encourage the body's own natural healing ability. By unblocking the congestion, energy can flow freely and good health will be restored. This is called a state of homeostasis.

USING THIS BOOK

For simplicity the terms "practitioner" and "client" are used to denote the person giving and the person receiving a reflexology treatment. A reflexologist's main "tools" are his or her hands used in conjunction with "maps" of the hands and feet which relate reflex points to various parts of the

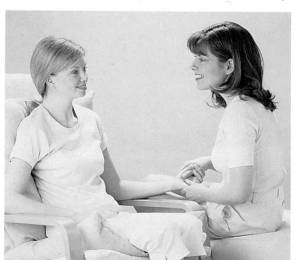

body. You will find these in Chapters 2, 3 and 4, which explain the body systems. A reflexologist may work one particular system or cover them all in a full treatment.

Although the advice and information in this book is to encourage individuals to work their own reflexes to improve their wellbeing, it should not replace an appointment with a qualified reflexologist or a visit to your doctor for any undiagnosed pain.

WHAT IS REFLEXOLOGY?

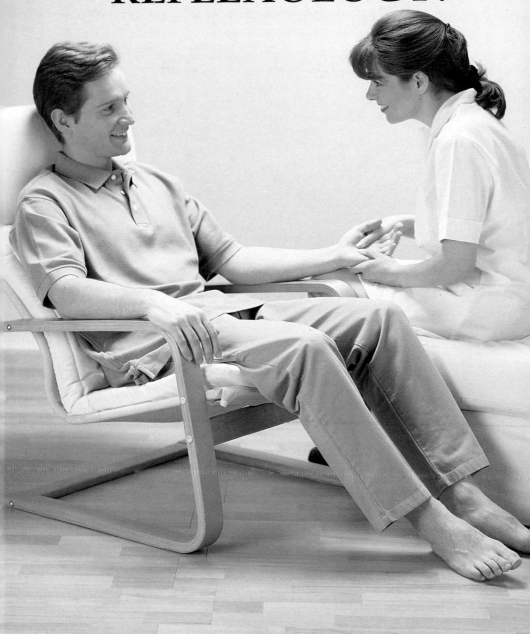

WHAT REFLEXOLOGY DOES

Reflexologists believe there are points on the feet and hands that can be worked on to bring about change within the body. The well-being of the client is paramount. Reflexologists should be trained to a high standard. Only those who are doctors have a licence to practise medicine. Some may have other medical qualifications, but generally reflexologists do not diagnose; their purpose is to work the reflexes to locate the sensitive points which may indicate areas of imbalance.

ENCOURAGING NATURAL HEALING

Reflexologists do not make claims to cure. Unless they have a medical qualification which allows them to, they do not prescribe or adjust medication. They do not recommend nutritional supplements unless they are also nutritionists. In some Eastern countries short sticks or probes are used to stimulate the reflexes, but this is not common practice in Western Europe or the United States. Nor do reflexologists give unqualified advice. Their intention is to encourage the body's natural healing ability.

You do not have to be unwell, however, to enjoy reflexology – there are many benefits to be gained from experiencing this gentle therapy.

RELAXATION

Reflexology reduces stress in the body and releases negative tension. Many physical problems can be the result of outside pressure and tension. During a treatment, which lasts from 45 minutes to an hour, the aim is to encourage the client to relax. The muscles lose their tenseness and the blood circulates unimpeded, supplying the body's cells with oxygen and nutrients. The result should be a feeling of tranquillity combined with revitalization. When you are relaxed you function better. You sleep better, which gives you more energy the next day. This has a knock-on effect. You feel good, this makes the people around you feel good and daily tasks can be completed with enthusiasm.

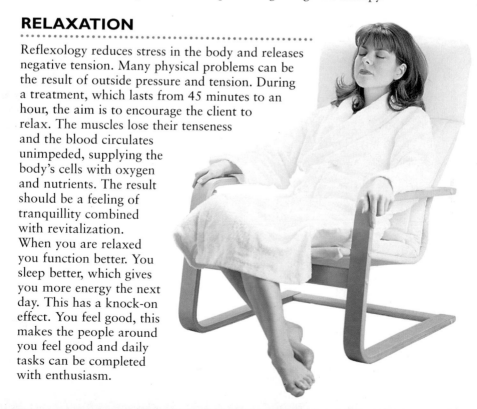

BODY FUNCTIONS

A full reflexology treatment on both feet or both hands will aid the release of toxins from the system. After a treatment people may notice that they urinate more frequently and have more bowel movements. Headaches and lethargy are also possible after a treatment.

PAIN RELIEF

When the feet and hands are massaged, as in reflexology, the body produces its own natural painkillers, endorphins, which relieve pain.

NO DRUGS

Reflexology is a non-invasive drugless therapy, which makes it acceptable to most people. The only tools are the practitioner's hands which use touch and pressure to help the healing process.

Please note

Before any reflexology treatment is given, a qualified reflexologist would do a full case history so the client's state of health is known.

For all practitioners, the basic rule is: if in any doubt at all, do not give a reflexology treatment.

WHEN CARE SHOULD BE TAKEN

Reflexology is a very safe, gentle treatment and can be used on any age group, from young children to elderly people. As with all forms of alternative/complementary therapy, there are times when certain conditions are contra-indicated or when care or judgement is needed.

■ First trimester of pregnancy: in first pregnancies and where there have been previous miscarriages or difficulties in the early stages, reflexology should not be given. In other cases, research has shown reflexology can have beneficial effects during pregnancy.

■ Thrombosis: treatment should not be given without the consent of a doctor.

■ Surgery: after recent surgery or where there is any internal bleeding, care should be taken. Reflexologists who work in hospitals are encouraged to work on patients before and after surgery to help the healing process, with the agreement of the doctor in charge.

■ Heart attack: reflexology is contra-indicated in someone who has had a heart attack. Wait at least three months to give the heart muscle time to recover, and the patient should consult his or her doctor before having a treatment.

■ Flu or contagious conditions: people with a high temperature, fever or rash generally do not feel very well. Stimulating their body with reflexology will only make them feel worse.

■ Elderly men and women, young children, very sick or terminally ill people: use very light pressure and shorten the length of treatment time.

THE ENERGY ZONES

Reflexologists work on 10 longitudinal energy zones that extend throughout the body. They believe that any disorder that upsets the flow of energy through a particular zone will interfere with the healthy functioning of other parts of the body in the same zone.

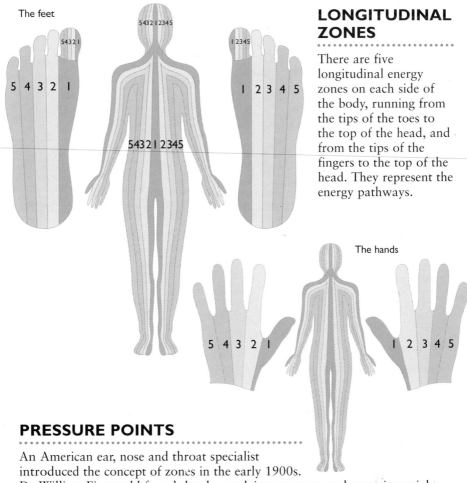

The feet

The hands

LONGITUDINAL ZONES

There are five longitudinal energy zones on each side of the body, running from the tips of the toes to the top of the head, and from the tips of the fingers to the top of the head. They represent the energy pathways.

PRESSURE POINTS

An American ear, nose and throat specialist introduced the concept of zones in the early 1900s. Dr William Fitzgerald found that by applying pressure, and sometimes tight bands or implements, around the tip of a finger of his patients, he could create an anaesthetic effect elsewhere in that zone – for example, in the arm, shoulder or up into the face. Dr Fitzgerald believed that a form of pressure point treatment was known in India and China 5,000 years earlier, but that it was perhaps set aside in favour of acupuncture. In acupuncture, needles are applied to a meridian or 'energy pathway' to relieve pain elsewhere in the body and to bring harmony to that pathway.

APPLYING PRESSURE

Fitzgerald showed that direct pressure applied to any part of the zone would affect the working of the whole zone. This is the basis of reflexology. When pressure is applied to the reflex points of the feet and hands the whole zonal pathway is affected; it becomes unblocked and there will be a free flow of energy to bring about a state of homeostasis, or natural balance.

TRANSVERSE ZONES

The idea of transverse zones was formulated by a German woman, Hanne Marquardt, who trained with Eunice Ingham in the US (see p. 5). These zones run laterally across the foot or hand and correspond to different body parts.

If you imagine your hand or foot as your body shape, you can see that the transverse zone for the shoulder is at the top, the zone for the diaphragm is in the central area above the waist, and the zone for the pelvis is toward the heel or wrist.

Recognizing the transverse zones makes it easy to locate the reflex points. The liver, for example, sits on the right side of the upper abdominal cavity above the waist and under the diaphragm. Therefore the liver's reflex point will be found on the right foot or hand between the diaphragm line and waist line.

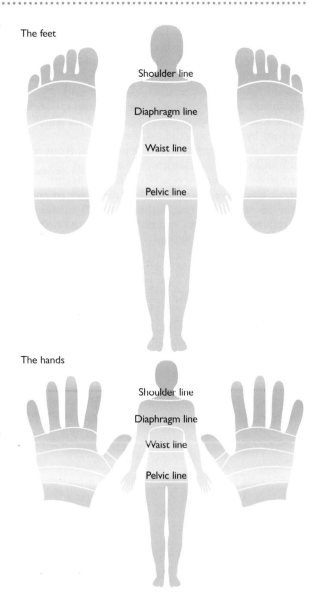

The feet

Shoulder line

Diaphragm line

Waist line

Pelvic line

The hands

Shoulder line

Diaphragm line

Waist line

Pelvic line

FOOT REFLEX POINTS

The diagrams on these pages illustrate the anatomical relationship between the body and the reflexes. In Chapters 2, 3 and 4 the body is broken down into systems, with explanations of how they work and where to find specific reflexes which may be on one or both feet. You will notice that many reflex points overlap each other and that some parts are located in more than one system. For example, the pancreas is both an endocrine gland and an important organ of the digestive system. When giving a whole foot treatment (Chapter 5), you work both feet to cover all the reflex points, which in turn stimulate all parts of the body.

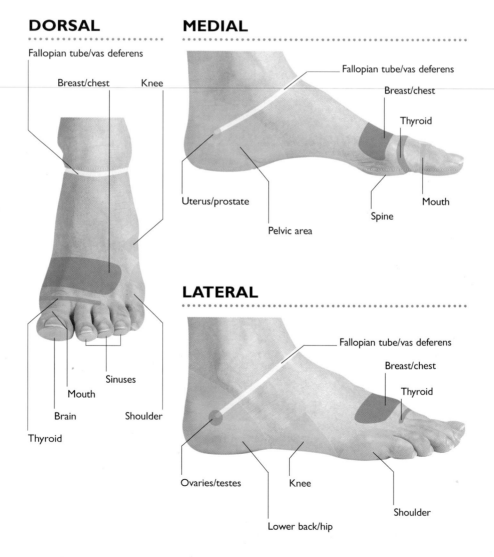

DORSAL

Fallopian tube/vas deferens

Breast/chest   Knee

Sinuses

Mouth

Brain   Shoulder

Thyroid

MEDIAL

Fallopian tube/vas deferens

Breast/chest

Thyroid

Uterus/prostate   Mouth

Spine

Pelvic area

LATERAL

Fallopian tube/vas deferens

Breast/chest

Thyroid

Ovaries/testes   Knee

Shoulder

Lower back/hip

PLANTAR

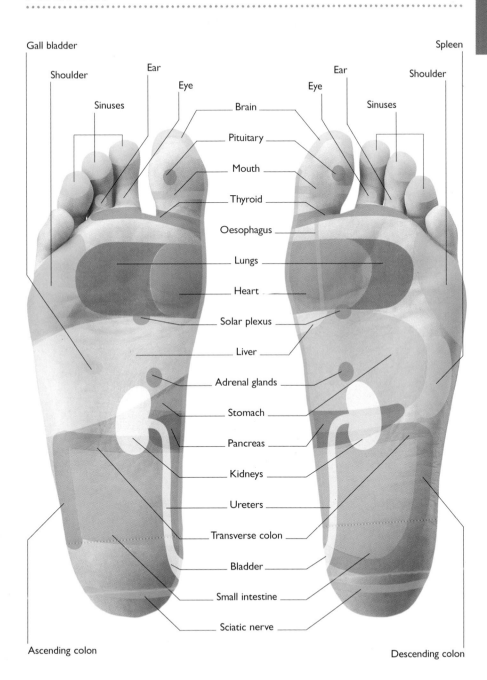

Gall bladder

Shoulder

Sinuses

Ear

Eye

Brain

Pituitary

Mouth

Thyroid

Oesophagus

Lungs

Heart

Solar plexus

Liver

Adrenal glands

Stomach

Pancreas

Kidneys

Ureters

Transverse colon

Bladder

Small intestine

Sciatic nerve

Spleen

Shoulder

Sinuses

Ear

Eye

Ascending colon

Descending colon

HAND REFLEX POINTS

When you look closely at the hands it can be difficult to see the relationship between the body and reflex points. Because the hands are much smaller than the feet, the points are smaller. It is a good idea to imagine the transverse zones (see p. 11) superimposed on the hands when locating the body part you wish to access, for example in the self help sections of each chapter. A whole hand treatment (see Chapter 6) is done on both hands to stimulate all systems of the body.

CONVENIENT TO WORK ON

There are many times when it is more convenient to give a hand, rather than a foot, reflexology treatment. For example, if you are working in a confined space, if the client is elderly or finds it difficult to lift his or her legs, if he or she is embarrassed about the condition of the feet or has a problem (such as athlete's foot) which should not be worked on.

DORSAL

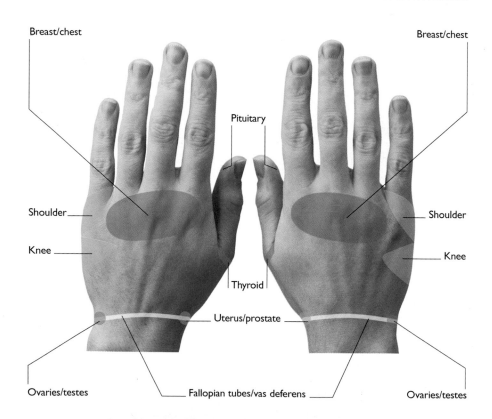

Breast/chest

Breast/chest

Pituitary

Shoulder

Shoulder

Knee

Knee

Thyroid

Uterus/prostate

Ovaries/testes

Fallopian tubes/vas deferens

Ovaries/testes

PLANTAR

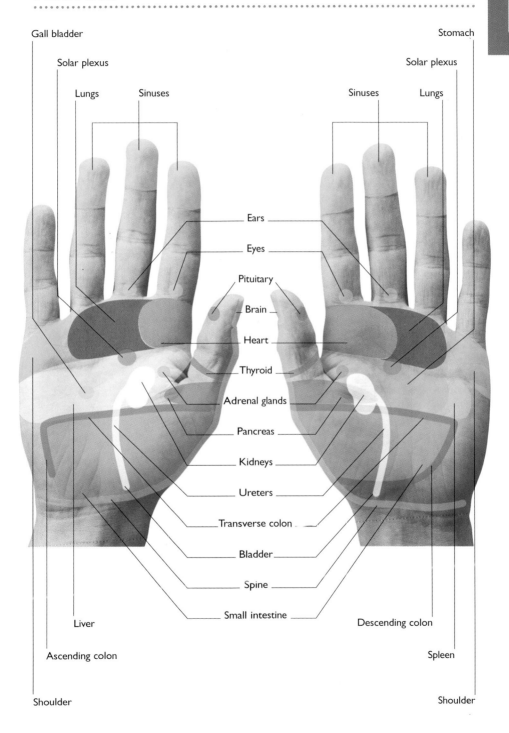

Gall bladder

Solar plexus

Lungs   Sinuses

Stomach

Solar plexus

Sinuses   Lungs

Ears

Eyes

Pituitary

Brain

Heart

Thyroid

Adrenal glands

Pancreas

Kidneys

Ureters

Transverse colon

Bladder

Spine

Small intestine

Liver

Ascending colon

Shoulder

Descending colon

Spleen

Shoulder

WORKING WITH OTHERS

All complementary therapies are complete treatments in themselves and reflexology is no exception. There are, however, times when clients like to combine reflexology with other forms of alternative treatments. Preventative healthcare is being seen as increasingly important, even in conventional medical circles, to society, especially now that so many people lead stressful lives, both in their workplace and home environment. Taking the time to learn how to relax and unwind has a rejuvenating effect on the body as a whole.

REFLEXOLOGY AND COMPLEMENTARY MEDICINE

■ Homeopathy and herbalism complement reflexology well. Homeopathy works on the principle of "like cures like", which means that any substance which causes symptoms can also be used to cure those symptoms. Herbalism uses herbs, usually in a liquid form, to treat the whole person.

■ Reflexology is good for alleviating spine problems, especially those related to the lower back and neck. However, there are times when it does not help a particular client, or when you feel that the client should be responding more positively. In such cases you should recommend that the person seeks help from a registered osteopath or chiropractor. These alternative therapists diagnose the body's misalignments by a method of sensitive touch and observation of the body's natural stance, appearance and posture. They use manipulation techniques and soft tissue massage; an osteopath also uses high velocity thrusts.

■ Bach Flower remedies are good to take when having reflexology treatment. The remedies, in liquid form, are prepared from flowering wild plants, bushes and trees and are used to alter states of mind or moods that hinder recovery.

REFLEXOLOGY AND CONVENTIONAL MEDICINE

Reflexology is becoming increasingly accepted by the medical profession. Many hospices, oncology departments and antenatal clinics employ reflexologists to work alongside the medical professionals. Many more nurses and midwives are training to be reflexologists so that they can combine reflexology with their medical skills.

It is important to remember that reflexology treats the whole person – it treats the stress that goes with the condition, rather than the condition itself. Using reflexology to support and enhance treatment can free doctors to allocate their own time more effectively. Some healthcare clinics employ a reflexologist to offer an extra service to their patients.

Reflexology gives a strong "feel good factor", which can have a major effect on patient satisfaction and recovery. There is evidence to suggest that complementary therapies in a medical practice can help reduce the drugs bill.

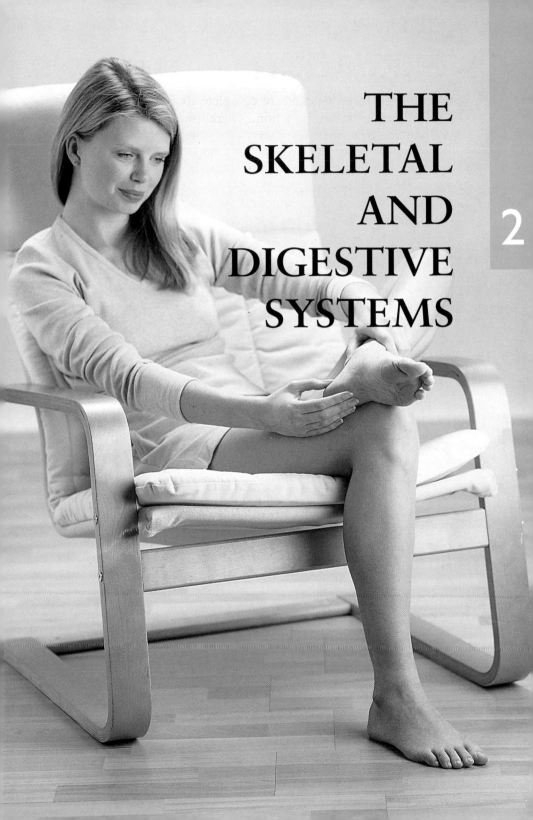

THE SKELETAL AND DIGESTIVE SYSTEMS

2

SKELETAL SYSTEM

The skeleton is made up of 206 bones, along with cartilage and numerous ligaments. The bones are classified as long, short, flat or irregular. The long bones, especially those of the limbs, are operated by the muscles to act as levers and thus allow movement. The most unusual bones are sesamoid, formed within a tendon, the best example of which is the patella in the knee. Bones have a strong outer layer and a softer inner layer, the marrow. The skeleton gives you shape, supports the body and protects vital organs, such as the heart and lungs.

2

THE VERTEBRAL COLUMN

Supporting the trunk, the bones of the vertebral column provide secure anchorage for the muscles and act as mechanical levers. Blood is formed in the bone marrow. To maintain healthy bones, it is essential to have a balanced diet with adequate amounts of protein, calcium and vitamins, particularly vitamin D.

THE SPINE

The spine is made up of 33 individual vertebrae: 7 in the neck (cervical); 12 in the chest area (thoracic); 5 lumbar (lower spine); 5 fused together to form the pelvic girdle; and 4 fused to make the tail part of the spine (the coccyx).

The lumbosacral area describes the bones of the lumbar spine and the sacrum, the bone at the back of the pelvis.

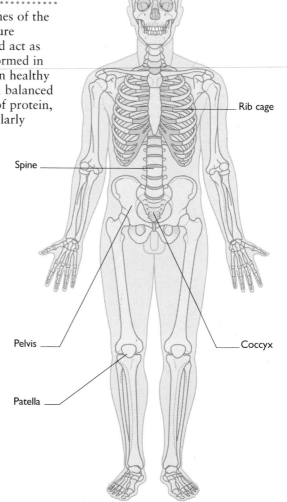

Skull or cranium

Rib cage

Spine

Pelvis

Patella

Coccyx

REFLEX POINTS

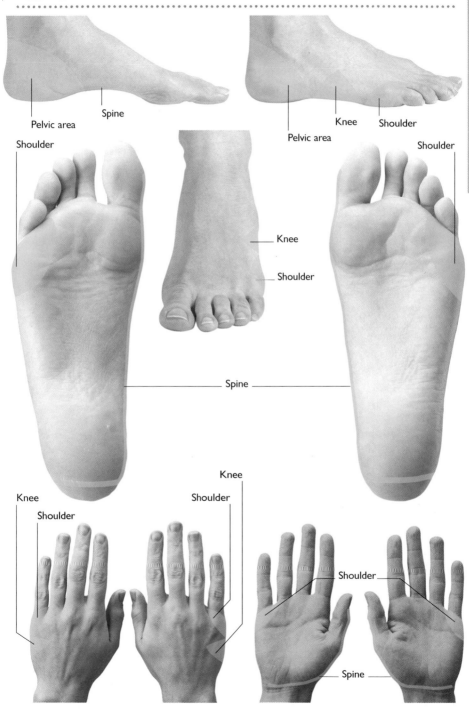

2

Spine

Pelvic area

Knee   Shoulder

Pelvic area

Shoulder

Shoulder

Knee

Shoulder

Spine

Knee

Knee   Shoulder

Shoulder

Shoulder

Spine

WORKING THE SYSTEM

When working the reflex points for the spine, it is important to remember you are stimulating the reflex points for the spinal cord which, with the cranial nerves in the skull, transmits messages to and from the brain. There are 43 pairs of nerves, 12 pairs from the skull and 31 pairs leaving the spinal cord at regular intervals between the vertebrae. If you have just five minutes to spare, it is beneficial to work these areas of the hand and foot as it will work the whole body.

SPINE

By working the spinal reflexes, particularly of the lumbosacral area, you stimulate the nerves and the blood supply to the area to relax the muscles.

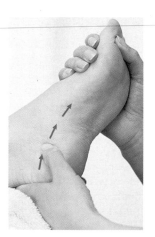

1 With the foot relaxed slightly outward and supported around the metatarsals and under the heel, slide your thumb up toward the toes. Use on/off pressure and rotate on any point which feels tender.

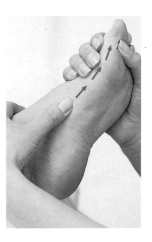

2 When the thumb movement becomes uncomfortable, change the hand position. Continue to slide the thumb along the bony curve of the foot to the top of the big toe, using on/off pressure. These reflex points relate to the thoracic and cervical regions of the spine.

HIP

In the pelvic region of the body, hips provide essential support for the frame. The cartilage at the end of the bones is vulnerable to wear and tear. Work the area on both feet to stimulate the synovial fluid in the joints.

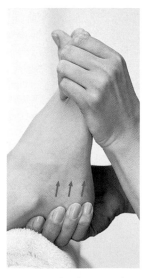

Support the foot at the toes and use your fingers, supporting the heel, to press and slide toward the ankle.

KNEE

Over the years the knee can be badly affected by too much kneeling or sports or carrying too much body weight, which puts extra strain on the kneecap.

Support the foot at the top. Run the fingers of your other hand down the lateral aspect to a knobbly protusion. Work below this, using on/off pressure, moving toward the instep.

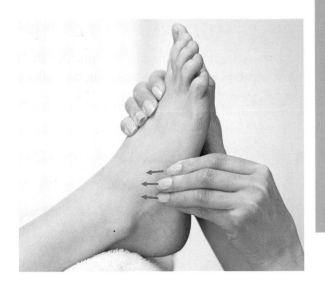

2

SHOULDER

The ball-and-socket joints of the shoulders, helped by a network of muscles, allow amazing flexibility. A good blood supply to the area prevents stiffness setting in when the body is inactive for long periods of time.

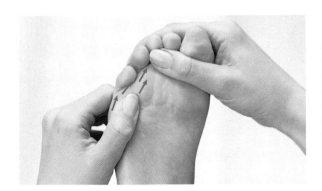

I To stimulate the plantar aspect, support the foot at the toes. Slide your thumb gradually up the lateral side between the diaphragm and shoulder lines using on/off pressure. Repeat using slightly firmer pressure.

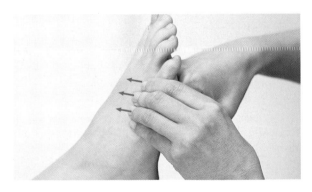

2 To work the reflex on the dorsal aspect, make a fist to support the foot and with the fingers of the other hand press, lift and slide from the lateral side toward the centre of the foot.

SELF HELP

The skeletal system needs a constant blood supply to keep muscles and nerves functioning well. By working the reflex points on your hands you can encourage healing in common problem areas. You should always seek medical help for undiagnosed or sudden pain in the back.

SYMPTOMS	TIPS
■ Back muscle spasm. ■ Pain that radiates from the back, down the lower leg (called sciatica). ■ Tingling sensations or numbness, either in both legs or just one. ■ Feeling of weakness in the legs.	■ Always bend from the knees when lifting any object. ■ Wear flat or low-heeled shoes. ■ Sleep on a firm mattress. ■ Do exercises that strengthen the abdominal and back muscles. ■ Lose weight if you're too heavy for height and frame. ■ Avoid sitting too long in the same position. ■ Add essential oils of rosemary or marjoram to a warm, not hot, bath. ■ Try gentle massage.

LOW BACK PAIN

The lumbosacral part of the spine carries most of your weight. It is the area that causes many sufferers from back pain most discomfort and lost working days. The typical symptoms are shown in the box above.

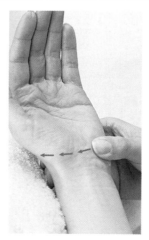

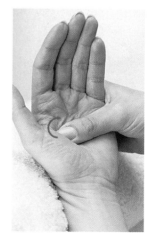

1 Use on/off pressure from outer to inner wrist to stimulate blood circulation to the lower back. Repeat 3 times.

2 Work the adrenal reflex to suppress inflammation. Rotate on the point using gentle pressure.

2

OSTEO-ARTHRITIS

This is thought to be a degenerative condition that develops as a result of wear and tear of the cartilage in joints. Without the protection of the cartilage, which provides a smooth surface for bones to glide over, the bones rub together. The parts most affected are knees, hips, spine, feet and hands.

SYMPTOMS

- Stiffness in the joint.

- Swelling and redness in the area that is affected.

- Pain on movement.

URIC ACID BUILD UP

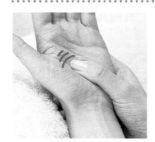

The kidneys help flush out impurities such as uric acid which form crystals in the joints. To work the reflex, creep the thumb in zones 2 and 3, using gentle on/off pressure.

TIPS

- Try to reach and keep to your ideal weight.

- Take regular gentle exercise, such as walking or swimming.

- Increase your intake of oily fish – salmon, sardines, mackerel. Eat wholegrain cereals, fresh vegetables and fruit daily. Include ginger and celery in your diet – their anti-inflammatory properties may help.

KNEE

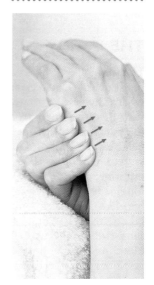

Work on the knee reflex to improve blood flow to the area. Press, lift and slide your fingers from the lateral aspect toward the mid-back, of the hand. Use gentle pressure.

FROZEN SHOULDER

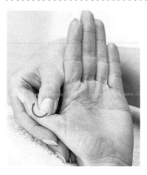

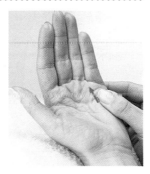

1 Stimulate the spine reflex to encourage nerve function and improve muscles tone.

2 Work the shoulder reflex with gentle massage along the lateral aspect in zone 5.

CONSTIPATION

The food you eat is processed by the body over a period of 12 to 24 hours. If there is not sufficient liquid going through the system at this time the waste becomes hard and is unable to move along the colon to be expelled. This causes the uncomfortable and sometimes painful feeling of constipation.

SYMPTOMS

■ Irregular bowel movements.

■ Difficulty in passing faeces.

■ Faeces are dry and hard.

■ Possible development of haemorrhoids because of straining.

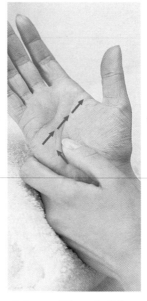

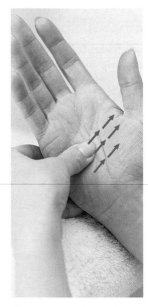

1 Press, lift and slide up the ascending reflex and across the transverse colon reflex.

2 Massage the reflexes of the small intestine and colon to encourage movement within.

TIPS

■ Drink plenty of fluids every day, plain water especially.

■ Take regular exercise.

■ Eat plenty of fresh fruit and vegetables every day.

■ Eat wholegrain cereals and wholemeal bread.

■ Avoid refined carbohydrates (sugar, bought biscuits, cakes).

■ Avoid taking laxatives, which can become habit forming and also remove some of the nutrients and water that the body needs to function efficiently.

3

ENDOCRINE, URINARY AND REPRODUCTIVE SYSTEMS

ENDOCRINE SYSTEM

The hormones in the body are governed by the endocrine system. It is made up of ductless glands that secrete the "chemical messengers" directly into the blood stream to be carried to target cells around the body. Together with the central nervous system, the endocrine system is responsible for the complex activities of the body. Whereas nerves cause quick reactions, hormones circulating in the blood stream are slower to act but they have a powerful effect.

HORMONES

Hormones influence growth, metabolism and sexual and mental development in different parts of the body, sometimes at a distance from the glands that secreted them. The glands involved are: the pituitary, the thyroid, parathyroids, the adrenals, the pancreas, the ovaries in the female and testes in the male. Hormone levels alter throughout life.

A typical example of hormonal influence is the production of adrenaline by the adrenal glands as a reaction to stress to prepare the body for "fight" or "flight". It causes the heart to pump faster as more oxygen is inhaled, blood pressure rises and the pupils dilate so danger is easier to see. Hairs on the skin stand on end, the face becomes pale and the digestive system slows down as the blood is directed to more important parts, such as the muscles, to prepare for action.

3

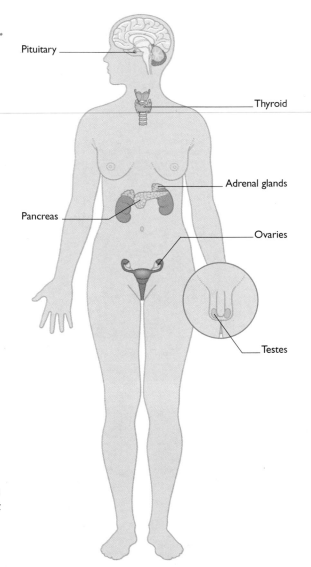

Pituitary

Thyroid

Adrenal glands

Pancreas

Ovaries

Testes

REFLEX POINTS

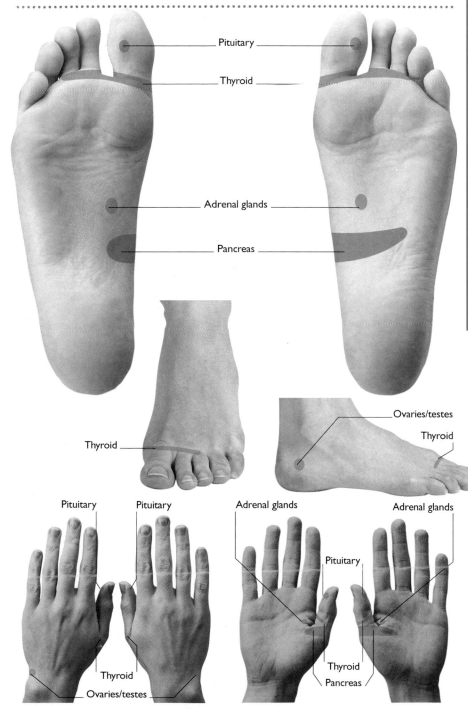

Pituitary

Thyroid

Adrenal glands

Pancreas

3

Thyroid

Ovaries/testes

Thyroid

Pituitary   Pituitary

Adrenal glands

Adrenal glands

Pituitary

Thyroid

Ovaries/testes

Thyroid

Pancreas

3

WORKING THE SYSTEM

The endocrine system is responsible for growth, metabolism and sexual and mental development. Regular reflexology treatments, working the reflex points of the ductless glands, combined with a healthy diet, relaxation and a positive attitude, can help to alleviate some of the imbalances that can occur at different life stages.

PITUITARY

The pituitary is considered the major gland of the endocrine system because it produces hormones that affect many other glands. It is situated in the brain just below the hypothalamus which provides the link between the central nervous system and the endocrine system and triggers the pituitary.

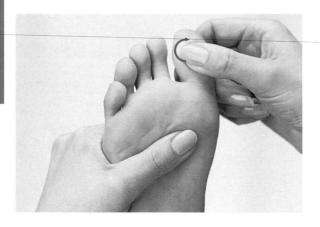

The reflex is located on both feet where the whorls of the big toe join. When working the right foot, support it with your left hand, apply pressure with your right thumb and gently rotate. The reflex is easier to locate when the whole area of the big toe (head) has been worked using the caterpillar walk.

THYROID/PARATHYROID

The thyroid gland is situated in front of the trachea, or windpipe. It produces the hormones thyroxine, responsible for metabolism, and calcitonin which helps balance blood calcium levels. Calcitonin works with parathormone, produced by the four tiny parathyroid glands situated behind the thyroid, to balance calcium levels in blood.

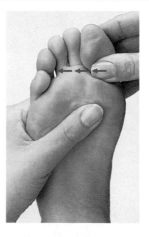

The reflexes for these glands are located where the big toe and second and third toes join the ball of the foot, on both feet. When working the right foot, support it at the top and with your right thumb press, lift and slide from the medial to lateral aspect, across zones 1 to 3.

PANCREAS

The gland that produces insulin and glucagon, which together balance the blood's sugar level, and secretes pancreatic juice into the duodenum, is the pancreas. It lies behind the stomach in the abdominal cavity. The reflex points are located on both feet – the right has the head of the gland, and the left has the body and tail.

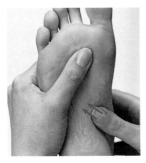

1 To work the right foot, support it with your left hand and with your right thumb massage the area just above and across the waist line of zone 1.

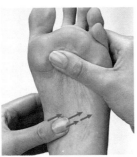

2 To work the left foot, support it with your right hand and use your left thumb to work from the medial aspect to the lateral, across zones 1 to 3, slightly above the waist area.

OVARIES/TESTES

Ovaries are the female sex glands at the end of the Fallopian tubes which produce oestrogen, progesterone and ova (eggs). Testes, the male sex glands, produce testosterone. They hang outside the body in the scrotum.

The reflex for both is on the outside of the heel. Use your finger to rotate on this area.

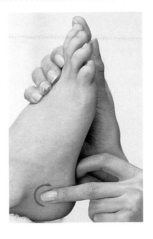

ADRENALS

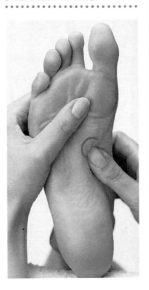

3

An adrenal gland sits at the top of each kidney. They are the stress glands and have two layers. The inner, the medulla, prepares the body for flight or fight by increasing the flow of blood to the muscles, heart and lungs. The outer layer, the cortex, produces cortico-steroids which help suppress inflammation and regulate the amounts of sugar, salt and water in the body.

To work the reflex, first on the left foot, then the right, flex the foot back and support it well. Move your thumb until you feel an area that is hard or tight and rotate on it with gentle pressure.

SELF HELP

The aims of working the reflexes of the endocrine system are to balance the glands and the hormones, and to encourage calm and a feeling of relaxation. Stimulating female hormones helps ease breast congestion and also rids the body of retained fluid, a problem during the menstrual cycle and at the menopause.

LETHARGY

When you have the feeling that you have to drag yourself to do something, that everything exhausts you, the energy lines of your body need unblocking. The reflex points to work on are the pituitary and thyroid.

SYMPTOMS

- Feeling tired all the time, even on waking up in the morning.

- Lack of interest in people or places.

- General lack of energy.

- Sluggish body functions (such as constipation).

TIPS

- If you are gaining weight and have little energy you may have a sluggish metabolism.

- Take up some gentle exercise – it doesn't matter what type so long as you stick to it and do it regularly.

- Change your diet so you lose weight gradually, not suddenly.

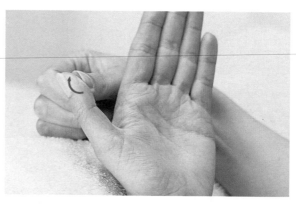

1 Locate the pituitary reflex point on the ball of the thumb. Rotate on the area with gentle pressure, then change hands.

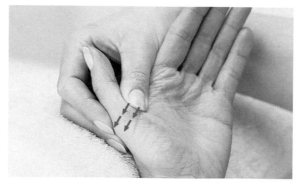

2 Find the thyroid reflex point on the medial side at the base of the thumb. Use gentle pressure to massage across the area, then change hands.

3

REFLEX POINTS

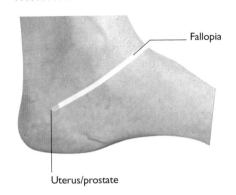

Fallopia

Uterus/prostate

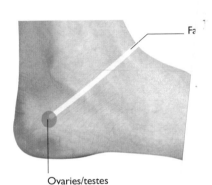

Fa

Ovaries/testes

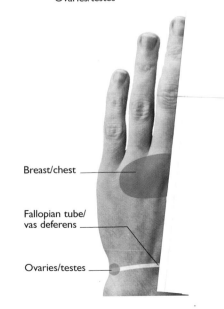

Breast/chest

Fallopian tube/
vas deferens

Ovaries/testes

SKIN PROBLEMS

The skin can erupt at various times of your life and can be a sign of hormonal disturbance. Since the skin is a major organ of elimination, it will be affected by a sluggish digestive system. Stress can also cause the skin to flare up, as can an allergic reaction to certain foods and substances.

The reflex points to work on are the kidneys and the adrenals.

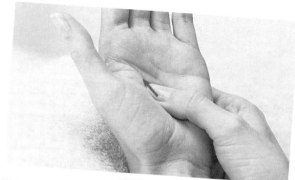

1 Work on the kidney reflexes of both hands to help flush the body of impurities. Apply firm pressure with your thumb to the kidney reflex, moving from zones 2 to 3.

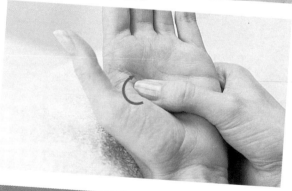

2 Apply gentle pressure to the adrenals (just above the kidneys), rotating on the reflex to stimulate production of the body's own cortico-steroids which help reduce inflammation.

3

TIPS

- Change the cleansing products you use in case your skin is responding adversely to one of the ingredients.

- Keep your skin protected – UVA/B rays and pollution damage the skin's layers.

- When choosing a sunscreen avoid any that can clog pores.

- Drink plain water throughout the day to flush out any impurities.

- Don't use exfoliants on skin that is red and irritated.

- See a doctor if a mole changes colour, becomes larger or bleeds.

REPRODUCT

The hormones of the endocr
reproductive system, p
reproductive system consists
tubes and vagina. The breast is
the female hormones, oest
reproductive system is made
testes, which all play their pa
The male sex hormone is test

FERTILE TIMES

Even with modern
advances in assisted
conception, a baby is still
made by the fusing of an
egg and sperm.

In a woman the ovaries
produce oestrogen and the
immature ova which are
known as oocytes and
were present in her when
she was born. During her
fertile years she will release
at least one a month,
called ovulation, from
puberty to menopause. She
may have started with
about 600,000 eggs but
only about 400 ripen.

In a man, sperm are
made in the testicles whic
hang outside the body.
This ensures they are kep
at a lower temperature.
man can produce sperm
from puberty and
throughout his life. Just
one takes about 70 day
mature after which it is
stored in a tube called
epididymis which join
vas deferens, or sperm
duct. It mixes with se
fluid from the prosta
become semen.

A PLAN FOR FERTILITY

The three body systems in this chapter are all interlinked and
conditions affecting one may have contributing factors from either
of the others. If a man and woman are planning to have a child, it is
important to work on the endocrine, urinary and reproductive systems.

HORMONE CONNECTION

The definition of infertility is the inability to conceive a child and carry it to
live birth stage. There are several causes (though, unfortunately, the most
common remains "unexplained"). Women may have an hormonal imbalance,
may not be producing eggs (ovulating), may have a blocked Fallopian tube or
problems within the womb. A man may have too few sperm or damaged
sperm, or his sperm may not be able to reach the egg to fertilize it.

Investigations and tests will be done to try and pinpoint the cause of
infertility. While these are taking place, reflexology treatment can work on
rebalancing the glands responsible for the production of hormones. In this the
pituitary is to the fore in both men and women. Working on specific reflex
points of the reproductive system can stimulate blood circulation to an area.
In men, working on the testes and prostate reflexes may help increase sperm
production and influence levels of testosterone.

Infections can be a cause of infertility. Working the parts of the urinary
system will encourage the elimination of waste and balance the fluid levels in
the body. Working the endocrine system will improve the production of
oestrogen, essential for reproduction during a woman's fertile years, and
progesterone. Without the right amounts of both at the right time a woman
will not ovulate, or produce an egg, and/or a fertilized egg will not implant
properly in the lining of the uterus.

Our bodies are fine machines which work well when all parts are attuned
to each other and are balanced. Keeping the energy pathways open will help
ensure wellbeing and good health.

ANTI-STRESS ACTION

The pressure of wanting a baby can put great stress on a relationship.
Relaxation techniques through reflexology will make a difference to the
attitudes of the people involved. A reflexologist will want to treat both
partners who are trying to conceive to encourage the healthy functioning of
their reproductive systems. A practitioner's advice might well be for a couple
to follow the information in this book to work on each other's reflexes to
bring about a state of calm.

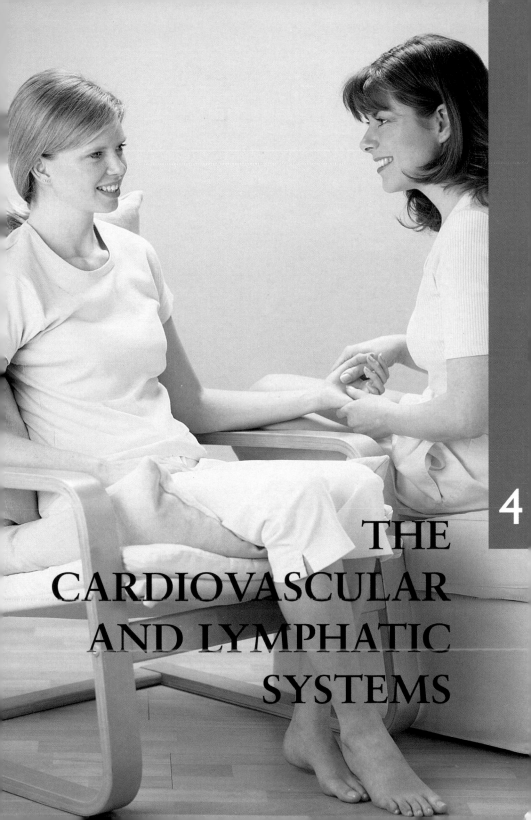

4

THE CARDIOVASCULAR AND LYMPHATIC SYSTEMS

CARDIOVASCULAR SYSTEM

The cardiovascular system is made up of the heart and lungs, which are connected by a network of blood vessels – arteries, veins and capillaries. Blood travels from the heart to the lungs, where it is oxygenated, and back to the heart for distribution around the body. Arteries carry oxygenated blood to the organs and veins return deoxygenated blood to the heart. The exchange of oxygen and carbon dioxide between the blood and the cells in the body's tissues takes place in the minute capillaries.

BLOOD

Through the powerful action of the heart, blood is continuously pumped throughout the body. The role of the spongy lungs is to keep supplying blood with the vital oxygen that it transports to all the cells while providing a way out for waste carbon dioxide. Blood is 50 percent water, 4 percent plasma, 1 percent white blood cells and platelets, and 45 percent red blood cells. Plasma is straw-coloured and contains fats, salts, proteins and hormones. Red blood cells, or erythrocytes, are made in the marrow of bone. They contain haemoglobin which gives blood its colour and carries the oxygen. Platelets, or thrombocytes, are also made in bone marrow and help blood clot to prevent unnecessary loss after damage, such as a bruise or cut, to the body tissues. White blood cells, or leucocytes, fight infection.

4

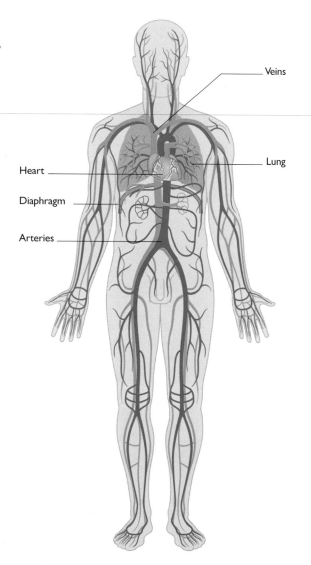

Veins

Lung

Heart

Diaphragm

Arteries

REFLEX POINTS

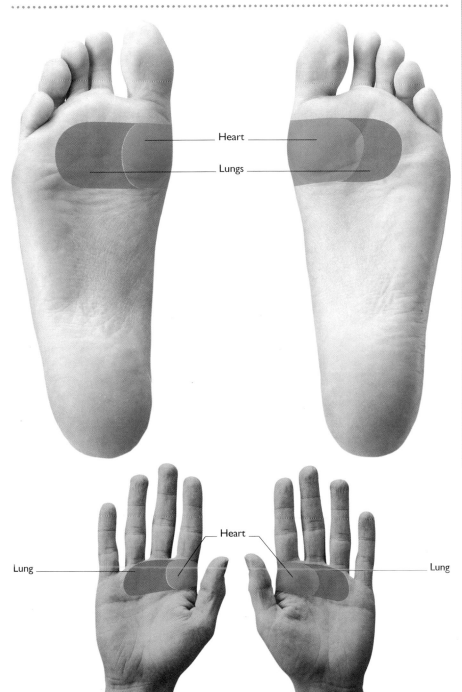

Heart

Lungs

4

Heart

Lung

Lung

WORKING THE SYSTEM

When you work the whole foot, you stimulate the cardiovascular system and influence blood flow, breathing and the body's immunity. The circulatory system with the heart at its centre links the three, carrying nutrients and oxygen to all parts of the body. Relaxing massage of both feet as shown here brings a feeling of wellbeing.

HEART

The heart is a four-chambered muscular pump. Although only the size of its owner's fist, it is the body's strongest muscle. Most of it is left of centre in the thoracic cavity and the rest is on the right – therefore the reflex points are on both feet.

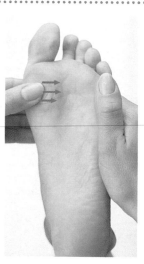

Start with the left foot, supporting it with the right hand. Use your left thumb to work the area above the diaphragm line, zones 1 and 2. Use gentle pressure and a sliding movement. Repeat several times.

4

DIAPHRAGM

A strong sheet of muscle that divides the chest from the abdominal cavity, the diaphragm is the chief muscle of respiration. It contracts and relaxes creating space for the lungs to expand into when inhaling, reducing it when exhaling.

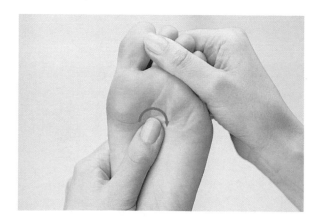

Relaxing the diaphragm will encourage better breathing. Support the foot at the top and place your other thumb on the diaphragm line. Gently apply pressure to the reflex point as you lift the toes to bring the fleshy ball of the foot on to your thumb. Rotate your thumb along the line, repeating this action.

LUNGS

The lungs are situated in the thoracic cavity, protected by the rib cage and resting on the diaphragm. Their main function is to exchange oxygen with carbon dioxide so that oxygen enters the blood stream and carbon dioxide is exhaled. This exchange occurs in tiny air sacs called alveoli.

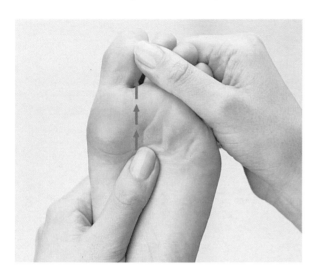

Hold the foot as if working the diaphragm. Use your thumb to apply gentle pressure from the diaphragm line up between each metatarsal bone, starting between zones 1 and 2. Continue in this way across to the lateral aspect.

METATARSAL KNEADING

This technique encourages the client to breathe deeply and slowly. He or she should breathe in on step 1, breathe out on step 2.

This movement is done as part of a whole treatment or for the purpose of relaxation and to stimulate the lungs.

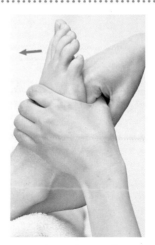

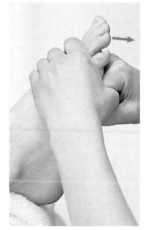

4

1 Make a fist with one hand and grasp the thumb of the hand supporting the foot. Push the foot forward gently but firmly.

2 After the client has breathed in, let the foot relax to the starting position. Hold it with your hand and squeeze gently.

SELF HELP

Exercise and diet are two of the easiest ways to help your heart and circulatory system stay healthy. Exercise strengthens the heart, improves circulation and keeps you fit physically and mentally. Eating less saturated fats in foods will prevent arteries furring up. Smoking seriously increases the risk of heart and lung disorders.

VARICOSE VEINS

When the valves in the leg veins which prevent the blood flowing backward do not function well and allow blood to collect, this stretches the walls of the veins, which can be seen on the leg as "knots". Varicose veins can be inherited, and women generally suffer from them more than men. Pregnancy and standing for long periods as part of a job can also be contributory factors.

TAKE CARE

■ Varicose veins should be treated carefully. They should not be massaged, since the vein walls, already stretched, may be fragile and may be injured by any pressure put on them.

4

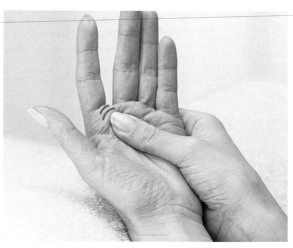

Use a gentle caterpillar on/off action on the heart reflex area to stimulate the circulation. Work from the diaphragm line to the base of the fingers.

TIPS

■ Avoid standing too long in the same position.

■ Don't cross your knees when sitting down for long periods.

■ Try to exercise regularly.

■ Cut down on foods high in saturated fats.

■ Wear good support tights.

ANGINA

When the arteries become furred up by fatty deposits, less blood is able to get through the coronary artery which feeds the heart muscle. The condition affects men and women during their middle to late years (women particularly at and after the menopause). Most at risk are those with a family history of the condition, those who are overweight, lead a sedentary lifestyle and have a diet that is far too high in saturated fats.

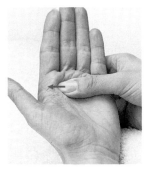

For angina, use sliding on/off pressure on the heart area to stimulate circulation.

TIPS

■ Change your diet to reduce fat and salt and include greater amounts of fresh fruit and vegetables.

■ Stop smoking.

■ Try to reach and keep at your ideal weight.

■ Follow a regular exercise routine which will burn calories, exercise the heart and help reduce stress.

■ Discuss cholesterol and blood pressure with your doctor and see if you need to change your lifestyle.

BREATHING DIFFICULTIES

The respiratory system is made up of the nose (including sinuses), mouth, larynx, trachea, bronchial tubes, lungs and diaphragm. This area is most susceptible to allergies and infections.

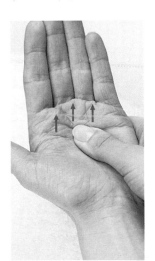

To encourage the lungs to work well, apply gentle on/off pressure on the reflexes. Work from the diaphragm line up between the metacarpal bones. Repeat with firmer pressure.

TIPS

■ Learn to breathe properly. Many people do not use their lungs to full capacity.

■ Breathe in slowly and deeply, counting to four. Hold your breath for a count of four and then slowly breathe out to a count of four.

■ Stop smoking.

■ Take up regular exercise such as walking or cycling – wear a mouth mask to protect against allergens or cold air.

4

LYMPHATIC SYSTEM

The lymphatic system is a secondary circulatory system which is also known as the immune system. It is a fine network that runs parallel to the circulating blood and its role is to protect the body. There are two signs that the body is fighting infection: fever, and enlarged lymph glands. The immune system's major organ is the spleen which filters the blood of waste and forms antibodies (immunoglobulins).

LYMPH

Derived from blood plasma, lymph is a colourless fluid rich in lymphocytes, cells that produce antibodies and protect against infection. One of lymph's primary functions is to provide a fluid environment between cells and tissues in all parts of the body. It drains through lymphatic tissue at lymph nodes, one-way valves in the neck, armpits and groin, that filter out bacteria, viruses and worn-out blood cells which may have entered the tissues as a result of disease or injury. The lymph clears this harmful matter before returning to the blood circulation at the thoracic vein. The lymphatic system does not have a pump (as the heart is in the cardiovascular system) and lymph is moved around the body by the contraction of surrounding muscle and by the valves which ensure it moves in the right direction. A reflexologist works the reflexes of the entry points of infection.

4

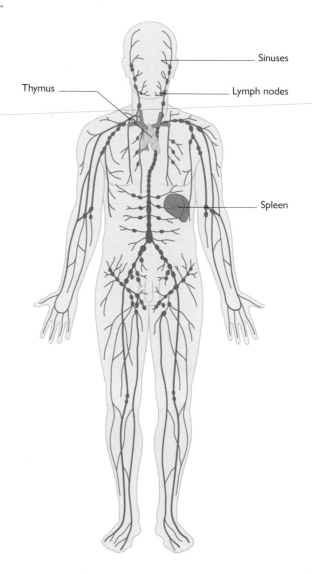

Sinuses

Thymus

Lymph nodes

Spleen

REFLEX POINTS

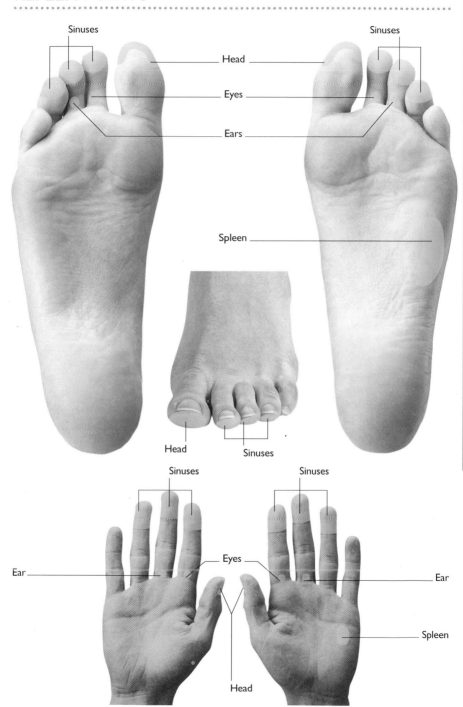

Sinuses
Head
Eyes
Ears
Sinuses

Spleen

Head
Sinuses

Sinuses
Sinuses
Eyes
Ear
Ear
Spleen
Head

4

WORKING THE SYSTEM

All the parts that make up the lymphatic system have one purpose: to filter out any harmful matter and protect the blood circulation. By working the reflexes of the system you increase the body's immunity to infection. The smallest part, the thymus, which produces T-lymphocytes, is stimulated when the heart/lung area is worked on (see pp. 68–69).

SINUSES

The reflex points for the sinuses are on the pads of the middle three toes, on both feet. The sinuses are affected when people have colds, blocked noses and hay fever.
You can expect your client to sniff when you work on these reflexes.

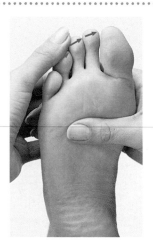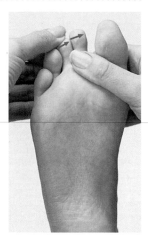

1 Support the foot and apply gentle pressure, starting from the lateral aspect.

2 Move on from toe to toe, massaging the reflexes. Repeat several times.

SPLEEN

This organ is situated behind the stomach on the left-hand side of the abdomen. It breaks down and renews worn-out blood cells and produces antibodies which help combat infection. The spleen also stores iron.

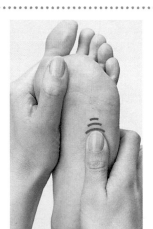

The reflex is on the left foot. Support the foot and use your right thumb to work zones 4 and 5, from the waist line to diaphragm line. A caterpillar movement, with on/off pressure, is effective.

4

ADENOIDS/TONSILS

The tonsils are a mass of lymphatic tissue in the back of the throat; the adenoids are behind the nose. Both act to protect the respiratory tract.

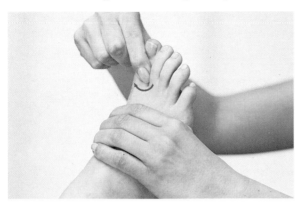

The reflex point is located between the big toe and second toe. Use your index finger to gently rotate on this point. Repeat frequently if the tonsils or adenoids are infected.

LYMPHATIC SQUEEZE

These two movements help the flow of lymph in the tissues of the feet. It is a gentle action.

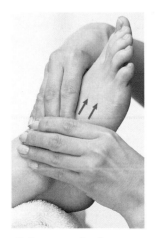 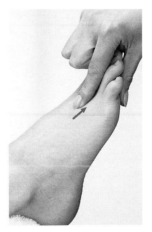

1 Support the foot with your thumbs and draw your crossed fingers up the centre, then up each side.

2 Press in between each metatarsal bone with your index finger, using your thumb as support.

LYMPHATIC DRAINAGE

This moves any fluid that has built up in the tissues of the feet causing swelling. Work the dorsal aspect gently, making long pushing movements with your hands, from the toes down to the ankles.

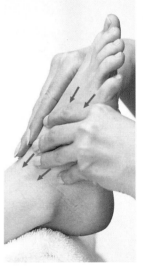

Support the foot with your thumbs and slide both hands together down the foot to the ankles. Lift your fingers and go back to the top. Repeat a few times. It should feel soothing to receive and you will see the fluid move.

4

SELF HELP

The lymphatic system is also called the immune system because it defends the body against bacteria and viruses that are so easily passed on from person to person. To keep the immune system strong enough to defend against attack, you need to eat healthily, take plenty of recreation and fresh air and sleep well.

COMMON COLDS AND FLU

These are the most common everyday illnesses which spread when people get together – at work and on public transport. Colds are viral infections which spread by coughing and sneezing, especially in confined areas.

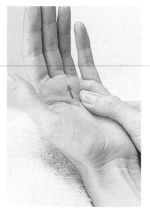
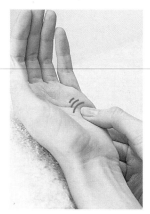
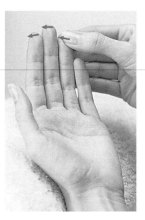

4

1 The lung reflex points are on both hands, zones 2 to 5. Press and slide from the diaphragm up between each metacarpal bone.

2 Use an on/off caterpillar movement on the spleen reflex, in zone 5 between the waist and diaphragm lines.

3 Use the thumb to compress the sinus reflexes on the first three fingers. Work one finger at a time and vary the pressure.

TIPS

- Take plenty of rest, to allow the body to recover.

- Use garlic and onions in your cooking – they have antiviral and antibacterial properties.

- Eat fruit and vegetables rich in vitamin C.

- Drink plenty of fluids, especially plain water.

- Use essential oils of eucalyptus and tea tree in steam inhalations.

ALLERGIES

More and more people suffer from allergic reactions to ever-present microorganisms in the environment. Hay fever is an increasingly common condition, causing runny eyes and nose, sneezing and sometimes wheezing. Working the head, sinus and spleen reflexes can help the body fight this invasion.

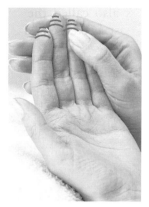 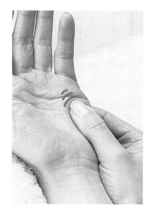

1 Use the caterpillar on/off movement along the length of each finger and the thumb to stimulate the head area.

2 For the immune system, caterpillar walk up the area between the waist and diaphragm lines.

RHEUMATOID ARTHRITIS

Unlike osteo-arthritis, this is an autoimmune condition in which the body attacks its own tissues. The parts of the body most commonly affected are the feet and hands, which can be painful to touch so care must be taken.

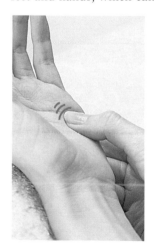 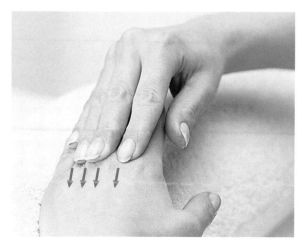

4

The reflex for the spleen should be worked gently to help the body's defence.

Lymphatic drainage is especially soothing when rheumatoid arthritis affects the hands and makes them swollen. Glide your fingers very gently from knuckles to wrist. Repeat several times.

BOOSTING IMMUNITY

To keep the immune system functioning at the level which ensures maximum wellbeing, it may be necessary to take steps to counteract the general negative effects of stress. These can be separated into three areas: behavioural, physical and emotional.

BEHAVIOURAL

Sudden overindulgence in smoking, drinking or eating can be a sign of stress, as can impulsive emotional behaviour which is out of character, and being unable to tolerate or relate to others at home and work.

PHYSICAL

Pains that are neither muscular in origin nor brought about by strenuous activity may be due to stress. Backache, neck tension, chest pain, headaches and nausea can all be the end result of stress.

EMOTIONAL

When stress goes on for a long time it can be emotionally draining. It can make you feel constantly tired, uninterested in everyday activities, unable to concentrate and cause you to have a low opinion of yourself.

STEPS TO STRENGTHEN YOUR SYSTEM

- Try to list the jobs you have to do and put them in order of importance.

- Learn how to breathe deeply and slowly. It brings oxygen-rich air into your body and helps to calm you in a stressful situation.

- Release pent-up energy through exercise, particularly outdoors where you will benefit from fresh air which will help you sleep better.

- Allow time for yourself.

- Take up a meditational pastime such as yoga.

- Have an early night after a long soak in a warm bath to which six drops of essential oil have been added. Choose from relaxing oils such as lavender, chamomile, bergamot or marjoram, but make sure you like its aroma or the effect will be counterproductive.

- When you have five minutes, sit quietly with your eyes closed and try to clear your mind by thinking of something positive and very pleasant.

- Walk by the sea, or in the country, and really look at the beauty that surrounds you: listen to the water and the birds and admire the colour and perfume of the flowers.

- Eat a healthy diet, with plenty of fresh fruit, vegetables and fish.

4

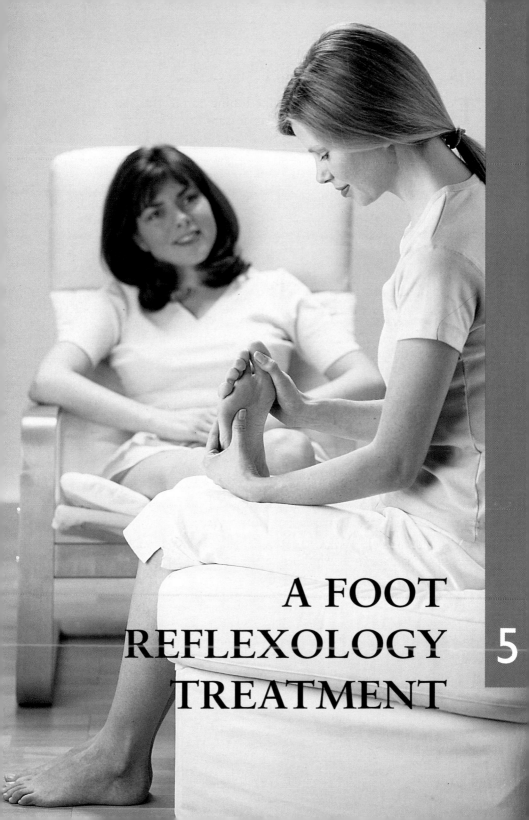

A FOOT REFLEXOLOGY TREATMENT

5

FULL FOOT TREATMENT

Ensure that you and the client are both comfortable. Cover his or her left foot with a towel and proceed to work the right foot following the sequence – from head to toes – in this chapter. When you have completed the right foot, wrap it in a towel to keep it warm and work the left foot, adding in the extra movements (see pp. 92–93). The closing movements (pp. 94–95) are carried out on the two feet simultaneously.

RELAXATION MOVEMENTS

The techniques shown on these two pages are designed to relax the client at the start of a session. They enable the practitioner to loosen the foot, which makes working the reflexes easier and is more comfortable for the client. One or more of the movements can be added in at any time during the length of the treatment. They should all feel pleasurable to receive.

SOLAR PLEXUS HOLD

Place the thumbs of both hands on the solar plexus point and use the fingers of the hands to support the foot around the dorsal area. Apply firm pressure and hold for a few minutes. This is the first contact with your client and it is important that it makes him or her feel secure in your hands.
Lift your thumbs, move them up the foot a little, press and hold.

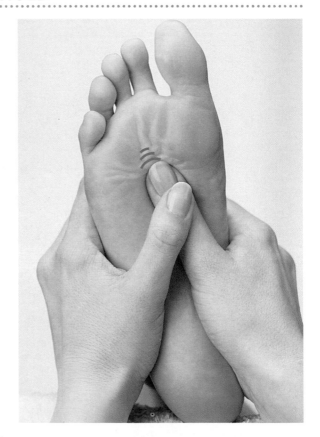

5

CROSS THUMB SLIDE

With your fingers supporting the foot, move your thumbs across the central plantar area keeping them parallel with each other. Work the whole area, keeping the pressure constantly firm on both the inward and outward movements.

SIDE TO SIDE

Place your hands either side of the foot around the metatarsal bones. Move your hands from side to side so that the foot rolls gently. This releases any tension in the foot and the leg.

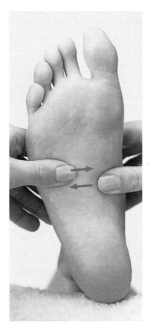
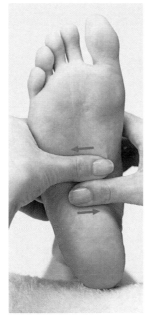
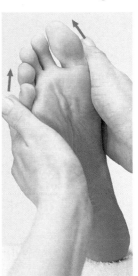

ANKLE SHAKE

Support the ankle bones in the cup of your hands. Gently move your hands forward and back, so that the foot moves from side to side. Do this for a couple of minutes to encourage circulation in the area.

This movement helps you assess how relaxed your client is. The more easily the foot moves in your hands, the more relaxed he or she is.

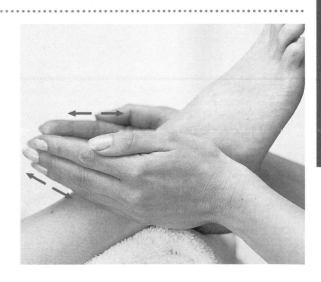

5

SPINAL REFLEXES

The spine runs from the brain down the length of the trunk and the reflexes for it are along the medial side of the foot. The foot needs to be slightly relaxed outward so you can access the reflexes. Support it with one hand around the metatarsals (fingertips towards the medial side) and the other hand under the heel (fingertips to the lateral side).

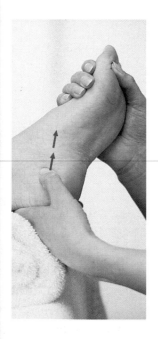
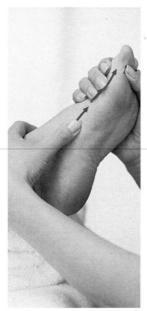

Using on/off pressure, move your thumb gradually toward the toes following the bony curvature of the foot. When this becomes uncomfortable, change your hand position. Continue working along these reflex points until you reach the top of the big toe.

If you come across a sensitive area on the spinal reflexes, apply a little extra pressure and release. Do this a few times or until the client indicates that the discomfort has eased.

TOE ROTATION

Support the foot with one hand and use your other hand to apply a little traction to the big toe. Gently move the toe from side to side, then rotate one way and then the other way. Do the same on all the toes.

This movement is very good for releasing any tension in the neck.

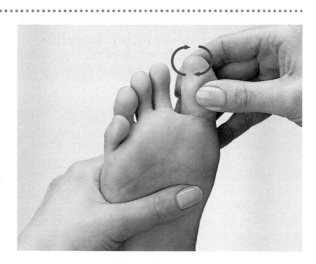

THE HEAD AREA

The toes represent the different parts of the head. The big toe has the brain (at the top), the pituitary gland and mouth. The tops of the middle three toes represent the sinuses. The reflexes for the eyes and ears are at the base of the first and second toes; they are small and can be difficult to work, but they are important for general wellbeing.

ALL TOES

Support the foot and use your thumb to apply pressure, moving from the bottom to the top of each toe. Start with the big toe (medial side) and move toward the little toe (lateral side).

It is beneficial to work these areas as they contain major points on the acupuncture meridians.

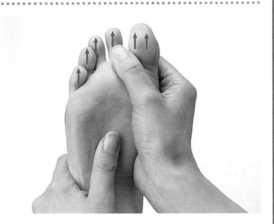

PITUITARY/HYPOTHALAMUS

The pituitary reflex can be found where the whorls of the big toe join; at times the area can look raised or puffy. Use the thumb to apply gentle on/off pressure to the reflex. If it is painful, gently rotate on the area.

Note: this is not an easy reflex to locate, but when you are working the whole of the big toe (as above) you are, in fact, stimulating this point.

BRAIN

The reflex is located at the top of the big toe (parallel with the nail). Apply on/off pressure with your thumb.

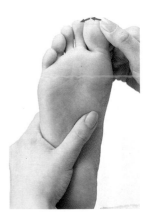

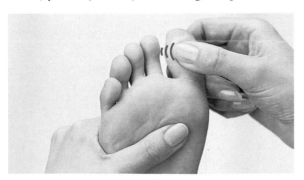

5

MOUTH

This reflex is found on the big toe, just above where it joins the foot. Apply on/off pressure with your thumb, working from medial to lateral.

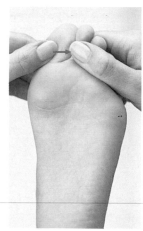

THYROID/ PARATHYROIDS

Both reflexes are located where the big, first and second toes join the foot. Apply on/off pressure with your thumb, from medial to lateral.

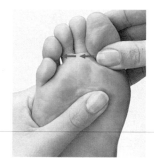

SINUSES

Find these on the pads at the top of the middle three toes. Support the foot with your right hand and use your left thumb to press, lift and slide across the tops of the toes, working from lateral to medial.

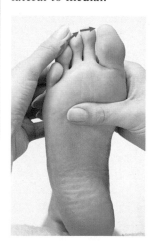

EYE/EAR

Find the eye reflex, at the base of the first toe, and rotate on it with your thumb. The ear reflex is at the base of the next toe along, and is worked as the eye reflex. It may be easier to use your index finger to work these reflexes on a very small foot.

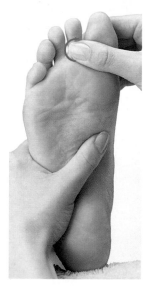

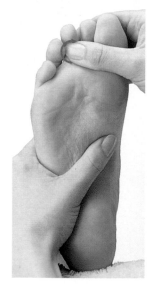

5

UPPER BODY

Start by relaxing the diaphragm: place your left thumb on the diaphragm line and support the foot around the toes. Apply pressure with your thumb while using your right hand to lift the foot and bring it slightly over on to the thumb. Continue along the diaphragm line.

LUNGS

Support the foot around the toes. Place your left thumb above the diaphragm line and press, lift and slide between the metatarsal bones up toward the toes. Slide your thumb to the right and repeat the upward movement between the other metatarsal bones.

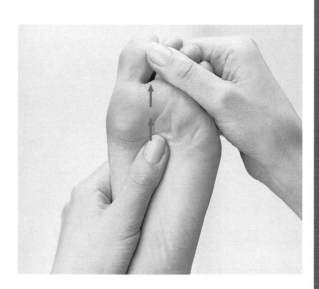

HEART

The reflex on the right foot is smaller than that of the left foot. Press, lift and slide from the medial side toward the reflex point for the lungs. Repeat twice.

BREAST/CHEST

Support the foot by making a fist. This will open up the dorsal aspect of the foot giving effective access to the reflex points. Place the thumb of the working hand in the fist which is supporting the foot. Press, lift and slide your fingers across the supported area, zones 1 to 5. Note that lighter pressure is necessary when working this area.

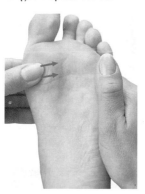

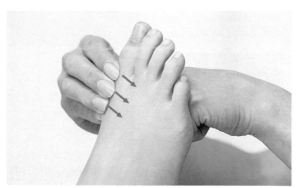

5

LOWER ABDOMINAL AREA

You will now work the area below the waist line which relates to the lower abdominal cavity. This area has the reflex points for the small intestine and colon. The reflex points for the urinary system are also located in this area, as are the points for the pelvic cavity and reproductive system.

SMALL INTESTINE

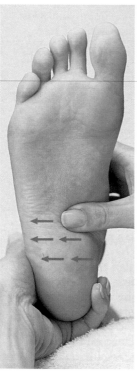

Use the thumb of the right hand to work the right foot, from the medial to lateral aspect. Press, lift and slide across zones 1 to 4, between pelvic and waist lines. Change hands and work area from lateral to medial.

ASCENDING COLON

Support the foot with your right hand. Starting from the pelvic line in zone 5, use your left thumb to press, lift and slide up to the waist line.

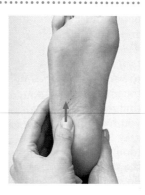

TRANSVERSE COLON

Press, lift and slide from lateral to medial on the right foot, below the waist line across zones 1 to 5.

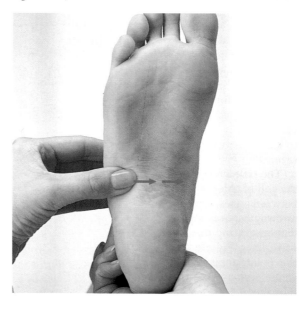

5

BLADDER/KIDNEYS

This area can sometimes appear to be puffy. Before working on it you might want to relax the foot (side to side, or ankle shake – see p. 81). Allow the foot to relax out to the side and support it around the metatarsals. With the right thumb work the area of zone 1, then move to the ureter (see right). The kidney is located in zones 2 and 3, slightly above and below the waist line. Use the on/off pressure of the caterpillar walk on the reflex.

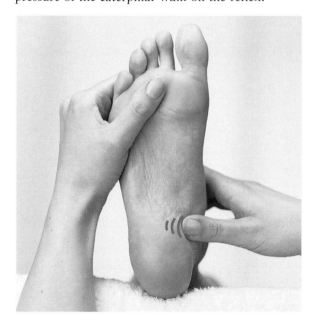

URETERS

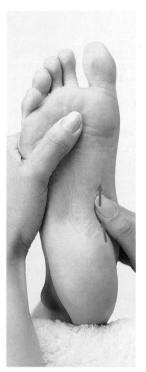

After working the bladder reflex (left), press, lift and slide your thumb up toward the waist line along the length of the ureter. This is located very close to the tendon. Now work the kidney reflex (see above left).

PELVIC AREA

The reflex is located in the inner heel area (and represents the lower back). Support the foot with both hands, at the top and under the heel. Press, lift and slide the fingers around the heel upward, to ankle level. Repeat several times.

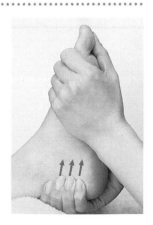

5

LOWER BACK AND HIP AREA

The medial, lateral and dorsal aspects of the foot are worked to stimulate the reflexes of important reproductive organs and those parts of the skeletal system essential to good posture, balance and movement. Use the relaxing side to side technique first, then continue as shown here.

UTERUS AND PROSTATE

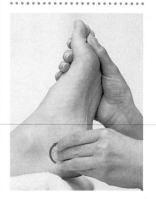

Find this reflex point midway between the inner ankle and the heel. The point can sometimes feel hollow. Use your index finger to rotate on this area, alternating the pressure.

BACK AND HIP

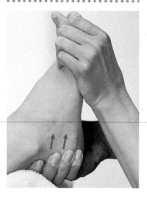

This reflex point is on the outside of the heel. Support the foot at the top, and place your other hand under the heel. Press, lift and slide your fingers up toward the toes. Repeat twice.

OVARIES AND TESTES

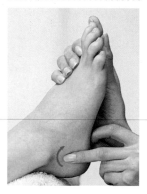

This reflex point is situated on the outside of the heel, midway between the outer ankle and the heel. Use your middle finger to rotate on this area, alternating the pressure.

KNEE

Support the foot at the top, with fingers pointing laterally. Run the fingers of your other hand down the lateral side of the foot to find a knobbly protrusion. Work below this area, pressing, lifting and sliding your fingers toward the instep.

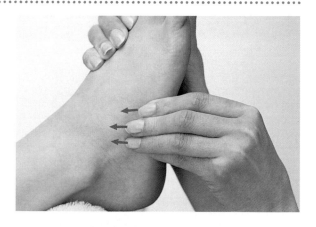

5

FALLOPIAN TUBE AND VAS DEFERENS

Encase the top of the foot with one hand and with the fingers of the other press, lift and slide from the uterus and prostate reflex down to the ovary and testis reflex. Now work the reflexes from both sides to the centre of the foot using slightly firmer pressure.

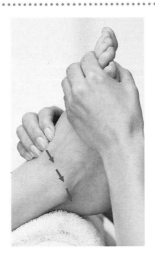
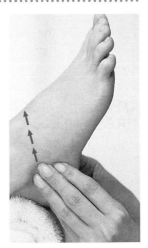

LYMPHATIC SQUEEZE

This movement helps the flow of lymph, dispersing any that has accumulated in the tissues of the foot. Support the foot with the thumbs and place the fingers of one hand over the other. With small movements and gentle pressure, draw the fingers up the centre of the foot. Repeat this on the lateral and medial aspects, from ankles to below the toes, then lightly press between each metatarsal bone, using your thumb as support on the plantar side.

SOLAR PLEXUS HOLD

To complete the treatment on the right foot, go back to the starting point – the solar plexus hold. You may find you can apply firmer pressure as your client is more relaxed.

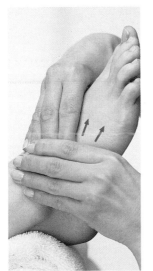
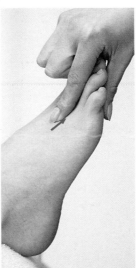
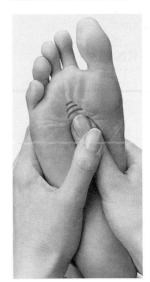

5

THE LEFT FOOT

Now work the sequence on pages 80–91 on the left foot with the changes shown here. Include the heart reflex before the lungs (p. 85). Work the stomach and spleen reflexes instead of the liver and gall bladder (p. 87). Stimulate the other pancreas reflex, the small intestine, transverse colon, replace the ascending with the descending colon (p. 88).

HEART

The reflex is mainly on the left foot between the diaphragm and shoulder lines, across zones 1 and 2. Support the foot at the lateral and dorsal aspects with your right hand and use your left thumb to press, lift and slide. Repeat several times.

SPLEEN

This important organ of the immune system is located on the left foot between the diaphragm and waist lines, across zones 4 and 5. Support the foot with your left hand and caterpillar walk the right thumb upward.

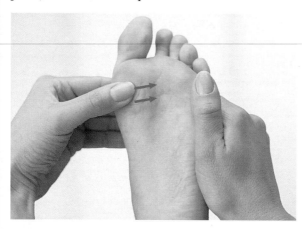

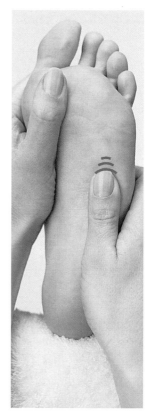

STOMACH

The reflex for this is mainly located on the left foot between the diaphragm and waist lines, across zones 1 to 4. Support the foot at the toes with the right hand and press, lift and slide your left thumb across the whole area, medial to lateral. Now change hands and work in the same way from lateral to medial.

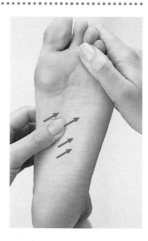

5

SMALL INTESTINE

Support the foot under the heel and press, lift and slide across zones 1 to 4 (medial to lateral) below the waist line. Change hands and work lateral to medial.

TRANSVERSE COLON

This reflex point is below the waist line, across zones 1 to 5. Support under the heel and press, lift and slide your thumb from medial to lateral.

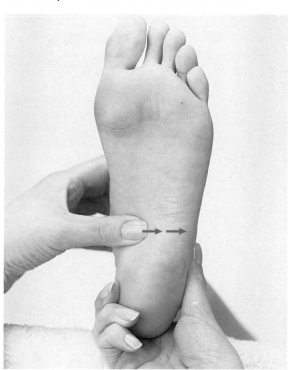

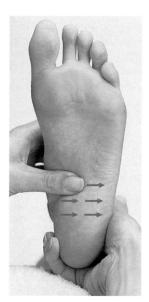

DESCENDING COLON

Support under the heel with the left hand and use your right thumb to press, lift and slide down toward the pelvic line. At this point continue the movement across the foot and then work up to the bladder reflex (which is also the rectum point).

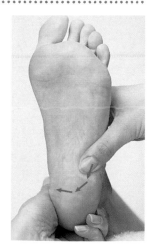

CHECK POINTS

Before moving on to the closing down movements which finish off the session (pp. 94–95), for maximum benefits take a few minutes to go back and work any reflex points that felt out of balance or were uncomfortable to the client.

5

CLOSING DOWN

When you have completed working all the reflex points on each foot it is time to finish the session so that you and your client both feel perfectly relaxed. The movements bring your hands in close contact with the feet, instilling confidence and reassurance.

SOLAR PLEXUS HOLD

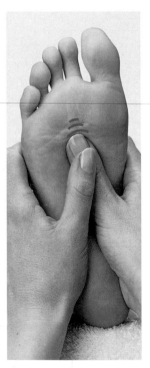

SOLAR PLEXUS BREATHING

This is one of the most calming movements of reflexology. Place your thumbs just above the centre of each foot and apply gentle pressure as the client breathes in. Release pressure as he or she breathes out, pause, then repeat three to five times. The movement should encourage the person receiving the treatment to breathe slowly and deeply. When exhaling, he or she lets go all negative energies and will be refreshed.

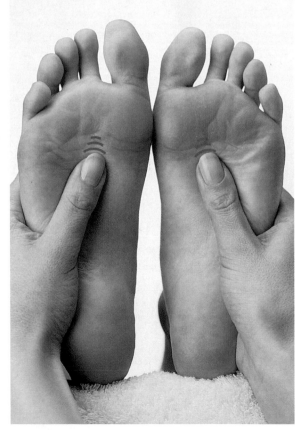

This is the hold for each foot, to start and complete a treatment. The thumbs are placed on top of each other to apply maximum pressure.

5

LEG PULL

Place your left hand under the heel of the right foot and your right hand under the left foot. Gently pull your own body away which creates a tugging feeling on the legs of the client and helps to release any tension in the lower back. Release and repeat once. Then place your open hands up against the soles and pause. You can sometimes feel an exchange of energies at this point – it may be felt as tingling, heat, a cool breeze. Slowly take your hands away.

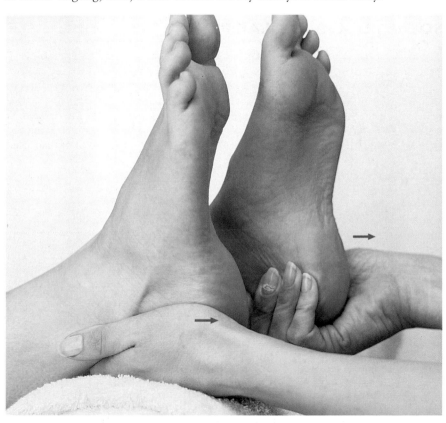

AFTER A TREATMENT

Encourage your client to sit quietly for a few minutes after the treatment as he or she may feel light-headed or, more commonly, sleepy. You may be surprised that you both feel thirsty at this point, so it is useful to have a jug or bottle of water nearby. It is most important to drink plenty of fluids to flush out any impurities from the body and help to ward off headaches. It is vital that the client listens to his or her body at this stage – sleep if feeling sleepy, drink if feeling thirsty. Have a light cover handy should he or she feel shivery. This is the body's way of coming into the natural state of homeostasis in which everything is working in harmony.

5

ASSESSING A SESSION

Reflexologists believe that the body is a unique whole and that working the reflexes is a safe and effective way of reducing stress and tension, improving blood circulation, aiding elimination and promoting wellbeing. You do not have to believe in reflexology for it to work, as you will see from your clients' responses.

THE CONDITION

Throughout this book, ways in which certain conditions can be helped have been emphasized. However, a reflexologist must keep in mind that the client needs to be ready to let go of the condition that is troubling him or her. The relaxing techniques and different pressure movements of reflexology help this process but the ultimate cannot be achieved until that person is ready to live without that particular condition. Such a person will start to get better and then stop coming for treatments.

ACHIEVING BALANCE

At the end of a session, it is worth reminding yourself – and your client if you feel it would be appropriate – that reflexology is a preventative health care measure as well as a pleasurable experience. Explain that you need to listen to your body, to consider why it has become sick, why you suddenly feel tired, are unable to sleep or concentrate. Like other pieces of machinery in everyday use, your body needs regular maintenance checks and the right sort of fuel to function at optimal level. You need to ensure your life is balanced in all areas, the physical, emotional and spiritual.

BUILDING CONFIDENCE

The more you use the techniques in this book, the easier they become and the more confident you will be as a practitioner. Working all the reflexes of the feet (as you have done in this chapter) and the hands (which is shown in the next chapter) works the whole body. This means, in effect, that it doesn't matter if you can't remember the specific areas you are working as long as you work all parts. It will help if you memorize the "maps" on pages 14 to 17 to visualize the body on the feet and hands so you can pinpoint different areas.

5

FURTHER TREATMENT

Deciding how many treatments your client will need can be difficult as individuals respond differently – some have a positive reaction immediately, others may require several sessions to feel results. As a general guide, most practitioners would suggest a course of six treatments, once a week. If the condition is acute – for example, a back problem – two treatments a week might be better. After these are completed, a fortnightly or monthly top up will be beneficial.

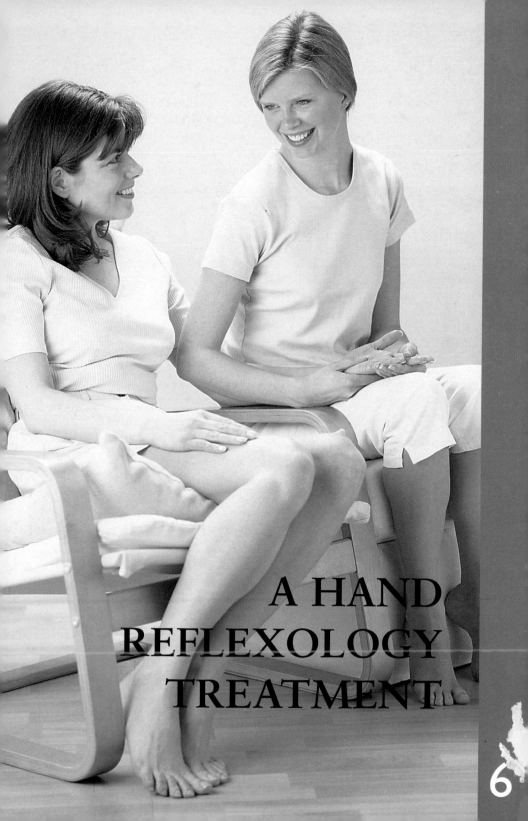

A HAND
REFLEXOLOGY
TREATMENT

6

FULL HAND TREATMENT

As with the full foot treatment, it is vital that both the practitioner and client are in a comfortable position, sitting either side by side or facing one another. Be careful not to twist your body or you will start to feel strain after a while. A hand treatment usually lasts about half an hour. Note that in this chapter either hand may be shown, but it is best to work the right hand first, then repeat the sequence on the left.

CROSS THUMB SLIDE

Begin the session with this relaxing movement to loosen the hand. Allow the client's hand to rest on a rolled-up towel or a cushion and support the hand with the fingers of both your hands.

1 Slide your thumbs past each other across the palm, keeping the pressure constant on both the inward and outward movements. Work the whole of the palm, moving backward and forward across the central area.

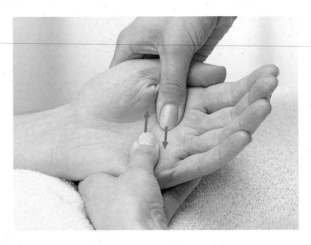

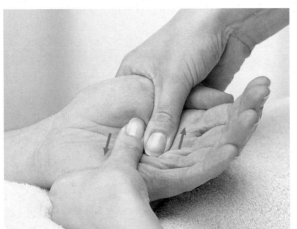

2 Repeat the action as many times as you like. It is an excellent relaxation method and makes it easier for you to access and work the reflex points. It should feel comfortable and be pleasurable to receive.

THE SPINE

The spinal reflexes extend from the heel of the hand to the top of the thumb. Ensure you support the client's hand as you work. For the most confident hold, place your hand underneath and bring your thumb alongside the client's thumb.

SPINAL REFLEXES

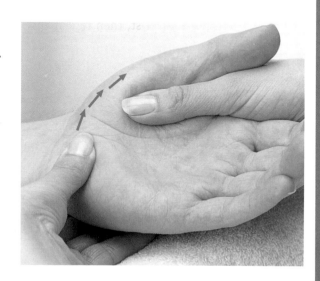

Use the thumb of your left hand to press, lift and slide from the heel area to the top of the thumb. Repeat at least three times.

You may need to change your hold a little as you continue working up the spinal reflexes along the side of the thumb.

SPINE/NECK AREA

This area is also worked on as part of the spinal reflexes. It is accessed most easily in reverse – starting from the top of the thumb and working down toward the heel of the hand (where the palm and wrist meet).

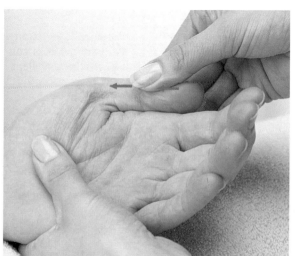

Firmly support the hand with your hand. Use your thumb to press, lift and slide along the length of the client's thumb to the heel of the hand. Rotate on any area that is uncomfortable or sensitive, taking time to massage it deeply.

THE HEAD AREA

The hands are much smaller than the feet so you will not find the same number of precise reflex points explained here. However, since you work on all the parts of the hand all the systems of the body are stimulated as you massage, apply pressure or soothe. Use your thumb or fingers to slide, press, caterpillar walk, pulsate and rotate, the last being especially useful if a reflex point or area of the hand reacts sensitively.

THUMB AND FINGERS

The fingers are much like the soles of the feet – very sensitive in some people. With the thumb they represent the whole of the head area, including the brain, eyes, ears and sinus points. When working on them, keep the pressure light.

1 Support the hand firmly and use your thumb to press, lift and slide along the thumb, starting from the thumbnail. Ensure you cover the whole area. Repeat twice.

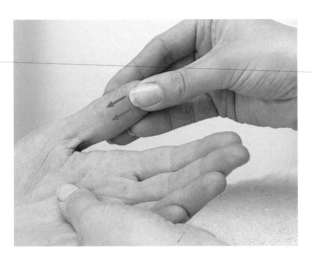

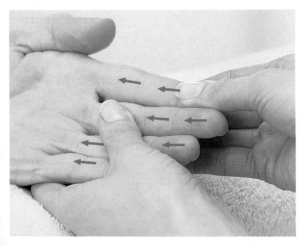

2 Work on one finger at a time, using on/off pressure and a sliding movement. Start at the top and work down to the palm, concentrating on each of the finger's three sections. Complete all fingers then work on them again, from the base to the tips, using the caterpillar walk.

SINUSES

The sinus reflex points are situated at the tips of the first three fingers and it is important to work down to the first crease of each finger. Press, lift and slide on each finger, then repeat several times, working at different angles. To finish, rotate on the tip of each finger.

Note: these are the points to work on clients suffering colds and hayfever.

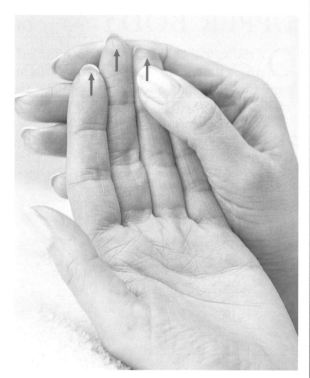

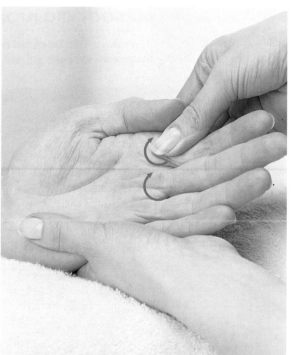

EYES AND EARS

The reflex points to these sensitive parts of the body are found at the base of the index and second fingers. Support the hand and rotate on each point.

BREAST/CHEST

Work on the dorsal aspect. Rest the wrist on a towel and hold the fingers with for support. With the fingers of your other hand press, lift and slide gently from the lateral to medial side. Repeat at least three times, then finish with a caterpillar movement.

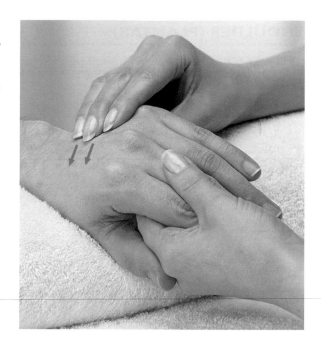

LYMPHATIC DRAINAGE

Hands, like the feet, benefit from being worked in this way, to disperse or reduce lymph in the tissues. It is also a calming and relaxing action.

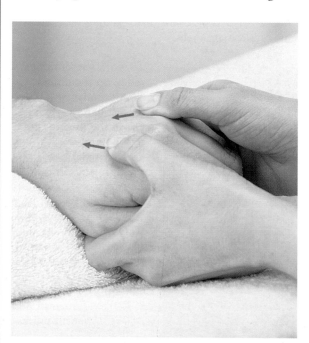

Use both your hands to give support. Now gently press and slide your thumbs between the metacarpal bones, working from the knuckles to the wrist.

It is important that this movement is done slowly and with light pressure. Repeat several times.

Note: extra care must be taken if the client has raised veins in this area of the hand.

ABDOMINAL AREA

The upper abdominal cavity contains the liver, gall bladder, pancreas solar plexus, stomach and spleen. The reflex points for the liver are on the right hand only; those for the stomach and spleen on the left hand only. In the lower abdominal cavity, the small intestine, colon and urinary system have reflexes on both hands. Working the whole area several times will ensure that all reflex points are stimulated.

UPPER ABDOMINAL CAVITY

Many people suffer with problems related to digestion and in giving a whole hand treatment it is important that this area is worked on thoroughly. To ensure that the treatment is effective, work from all angles and all directions. If a sensitive point is found rotate on it until it starts to feel better.

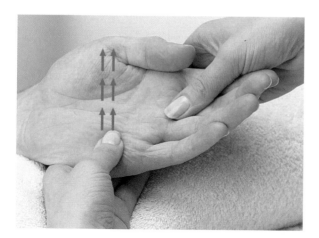

Support the fingers with one hand and work across zones 1 to 5 between the waist and diaphragm lines. With your thumb apply on/off sliding pressure, followed by the caterpillar walk. Rotate on any sensitive spots.

LOWER ABDOMINAL CAVITY

Support the fingers with one hand and work the whole area, from the wrist to the waist line. Alternate the pressure as you use your thumb to slide, walk and rotate over the area. Repeat several times.

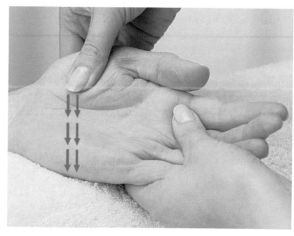

6

KIDNEYS

One kidney reflex is on the left hand and the other is on the right. The kidneys are organs of elimination and their reflexes need extra attention in cases of fluid retention, urinary conditions, skin and back problems.

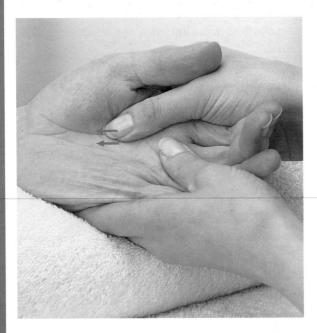

Support the client's hand with both hands and use your thumb to press and slide over the area between the more solid area (under the thumb) and the fleshy part of the hand. Follow with a caterpillar movement.

When working on the kidneys you also stimulate the adrenal (stress) glands that sit above them.

URETER

Continue from the kidney reflex, thumb sliding and walking down the palm to the heel area (where the hand joins the wrist). Working the whole area will also work the bladder reflex.

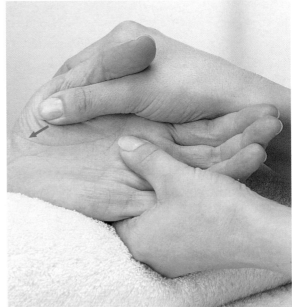

THE KNEE

Because of its vital role in mobility, the knee is an especially important joint. You rely on it throughout your life – if it gets stiff then you have problems. Keeping the knees in good condition requires regular exercise – they are not helped by long periods of sitting or not moving. It is a complicated joint and time spent working on the reflexes, on both hands, should be well rewarded.

KNEE

The reflex is found on the dorsal aspect. You may wish to do some lymphatic drainage (p. 104) on the area before working this particular point.

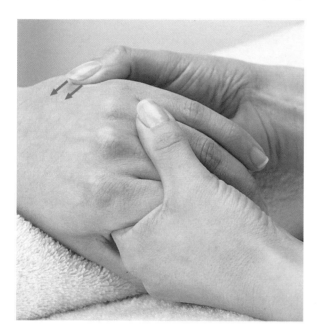

Make sure the hand is relaxed. Grasp the fingers to give support before working the lateral side of the hand, above the wrist. Use your thumb or fingers to apply on/off sliding pressure. You can also caterpillar walk this area. Keep pressure light and repeat several times.

PROBLEMS WITH JOINTS

The joints of the body are made up of bone, cartilage and synovial fluid, with tendons and ligaments ensuring connection to muscles. For movement, the muscles provide the force, bones are the levers and the joints are at the fulcrum. Bursae, fluid-filled sacs just outside the joints, can become inflamed. The condition is called bursitis, but you will know it by such names as housemaid's knee and tennis elbow, though neither housework nor tennis may have been the cause. Bursae act as cushions between bones and muscles or tendons and any sensitivity in the area may indicate the presence of inflammation to the reflexologist.

6

REPRODUCTIVE SYSTEM

The reflexes which make up the reproductive system are located around the wrist of the hands, on the dorsal aspect, either on the lateral or medial sides. When working these areas it is important for the client to be relaxed and for you to use light pressure.

UTERUS/PROSTATE AND OVARIES/TESTES

The reflex points for these essential parts of the female and male are found in equally accessible areas. They are worked on both hands. They can be worked together, as here, or separately (see opposite).

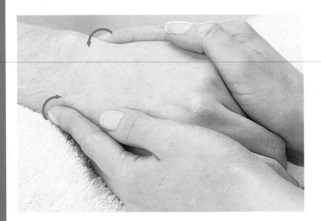

The uterus/prostate reflex is on the thumb side, where the wrist joins the hand. The ovary/testis point is on the wrist on the little finger side. Rotate on these points with your index fingers.
Note: if your client is menstruating, use gentle pressure, since working the reflexes can cause heavier blood loss.

FALLOPIAN TUBE/VAS DEFERENS

The reflex points for both are located in the same area, on the dorsal aspect of the hands, in a direct line between the reflexes just worked (above).

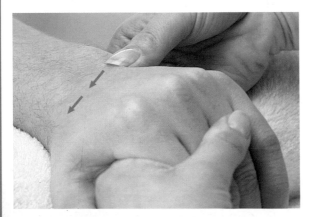

Support the hand under the palm, holding the fingers firmly with your thumb. Press and slide your other thumb from the uterus/prostate point across to the ovary/testis point. You can also use the fingers and vary the pressure with a caterpillar walk movement.

REPRODUCTION PROBLEMS

These are the areas to work on if your client and partner are having difficulty conceiving. Remember to work the right hand in the same way.

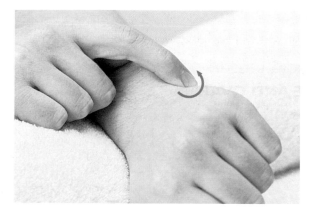

1 To stimulate egg and sperm production rotate your index finger on the ovary/testis reflex on the lateral (little finger) side where the wrist joins the hand. The reflex point can be felt as a little "dip". Use gentle pressure.

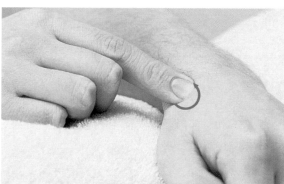

2 To encourage healthy functioning, rotate on the uterus/prostate reflex point on the medial (thumb) side of the hand. Use your index finger and keep the pressure light.

LYMPHATIC DRAINAGE

Support the hand and use your thumbs to press and slide between the metacarpal bones toward the wrist.

Note: once you have completed the full hand sequence on the right hand, repeat it on the left hand. Then move on to the closing down sequence (see p. 110).

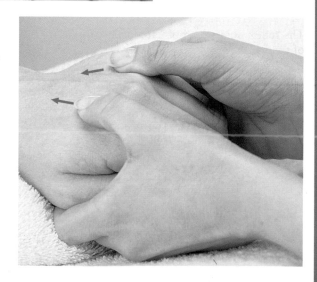

6

CLOSING DOWN

The movements are carried out simultaneously on both hands. But before you bring the session to an end, go back and rework any sensitive reflex points. Notice whether they are less sensitive when you repeat them. The closing down movements should be gentle and calming, so the client can let go of any tension. Encourage the client to close his or her eyes and relax completely.

SOLAR PLEXUS BREATHING

Allow both hands to relax. Locate the solar plexus points (just under the diaphragm line, between zones 3 and 4) and apply gentle but constant pressure. Encourage the client to take a deep in-breath. As he or she breathes out slowly, release the pressure but remain in contact. Repeat five times.

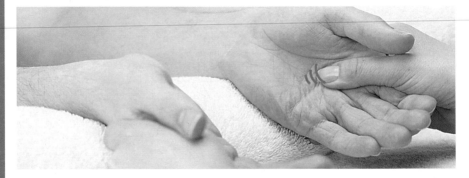

PALMS ON PALMS

Release the solar plexus point and allow your palms to rest on the client's palms. Hold this position for a few minutes. There are many sensations you both will feel at this time, all caused by the energy in the body rebalancing.

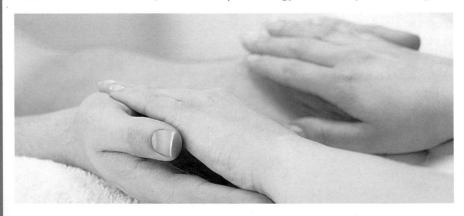

PERFECT RELAXATION

When a session has come to an end you and your client should feel completely relaxed. Allow the client to sit with his or her eyes closed for a short time as the body rebalances. This is the time when you should make a note of any imbalances felt during the treatment so you can encourage the client to work on these points at home.

TUNE INTO YOURSELF

After a treatment, the reflexologist and the client slowly return to normal. But during this time of relaxation you can review the treatment as a whole. Was it successful, did the client respond? You may want to discuss future sessions and what you would hope to achieve from them. Some people take longer to relax than others.

While the client is "coming to", you should shake your hands from the wrist to remove any tension and any negative energies. Now wash your hands, something you should always do after either a foot or hand session. Use a moisturizer to keep them soft.

AFTER CARE

Encourage your client to have a drink of plain water, not ice cold, which will help to rid the body of toxins and prevent any side effects of treatment (such as a headache). Remind your client to make a mental note of the way he or she feels a few hours after the session, and whether there has been any physical change. The unblocking of energy pathways and actions to release lymph can affect the body for several days after a treatment.

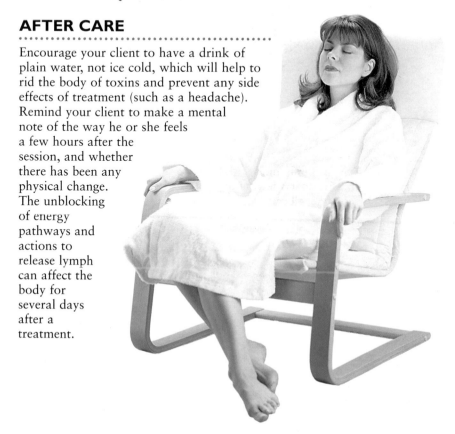

INDEX

ACKNOWLEDGMENTS
The author and publisher gratefully acknowledge the invaluable contribution made by Tony Latham who took most of the photographs. Other photographs supplied by Laura Wickenden, p. 20, and Andrew Sydenham p. 15.
Art work: zones Jenny Buzzard; reflex points Masumi Higo; anatomy Richard Tibbetts.